Culture in CLINICAL CARE

Culture in CLINICAL CARE

Bette R. Bonder, PhD, OTR/L, FAOTA
Cleveland State University
Cleveland, Ohio

Laura Martin, PhD
Cleveland State University
Cleveland, Ohio

Andrew W. Miracle, PhD
Florida International University
Miami, Florida

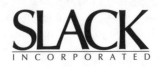

An innovative information, education and management company
6900 Grove Road • Thorofare, NJ 08086

The procedures and practices described in this book should be implemented in a manner consistent with the professional standards set for the circumstances that apply in each specific situation. Every effort has been made to confirm the accuracy of the information presented and to correctly relate generally accepted practices. The authors, editor, and publisher cannot accept responsibility for errors or exclusions or for the outcome of the application of the material presented herein. There is no expressed or implied warranty of this book or information imparted by it.

The work SLACK publishes is peer reviewed. Prior to publication, recognized leaders in the field, educators, and clinicians provide important feedback on the concepts and content that we publish. We welcome feedback on this work.

Printed in the United States of America.

Bonder, Bette R.
    Culture in clinical care / Bette R. Bonder, Laura Martin, Andrew W. Miracle.
        p. cm.
    Includes bibliographical references and index.
    ISBN 1-55642-459-0 (alk. paper)
    1. Clinical medicine--Cross-cultural studies. 2. Clinical medicine--Case studies. 3.
Clinical medicine--Social aspects--Cross-cultural studies. 4. Social medicine. I. Martin,
Laura. II. Miracle, Andrew W. III. Title.

Ra418 .B64 2001
362.1--dc21

                                                                        2001034471

Published by: SLACK Incorporated
                 6900 Grove Road
                 Thorofare, NJ 08086 USA
                 Telephone: 856-848-1000
                 Fax: 856-853-5991
                 www.slackbooks.com

Contact SLACK Incorporated for more information about other books in this field or about the availability of our books from distributors outside the United States.

Last digit is print number: 10   9   8   7   6   5   4   3   2   1

DEDICATION

To our students, our clients, and the many individuals who have shared their cultures with us, enhancing not only our understanding but also our lives.

CONTENTS

ACKNOWLEDGMENTS

The authors acknowledge their debts to those persons whose stories they have used and whose lives have instructed them in the relationship between culture and health. They also acknowledge the support of Cleveland State University, especially the Office of the Dean of the College of Arts and Sciences and the Department of Health Sciences, for providing them with congenial surroundings for the interaction that led to the idea for this book and then the work time and space to produce it. We thank Anne Fadiman for graciously allowing us to summarize material from her book, *The Spirit Catches You and You Fall Down.* (Ms. Fadiman did not write the summaries at the beginning of the chapters, nor did she participate in any other portion of the book.) We would also like to thank Wendy Schmidt, OTR/L, MBA for granting permission to include several photographs taken during her travels.

The authors are grateful to all the reviewers, who provided helpful and enthusiastic comments on an early draft of the manuscript. Their suggestions have greatly improved the breadth and clarity of what the authors have written. We express particular gratitude to Nadine Grimm, Program Coordinator in the College of Arts and Sciences, who contributed her great skills as an editor and teacher to the review of two stages of manuscript preparation. In addition, she participated in many helpful conversations about both the theoretical and pedagogical underpinnings of this work. Other helpful contributions were made by Tom Cinadr, who provided important additional Hmong references, and William McKinney, who gave us valuable critical suggestions. Thanks also to Adriana Pititto and her staff at the Stone Oven Bakery where we did some of our best thinking. We also thank Amy Drummond, Debra Toulson, and Joanne Ferrara of SLACK Incorporated for their enthusiastic support of this project.

Bette thanks her colleagues in the Department of Health Sciences, who have shared conversations about many aspects of culture and care, and Nadine Grimm, whose enthusiasm for this project kept her going when spirits flagged. She is grateful to her coauthors, from whom she has learned a great deal in an incredibly supportive interdisciplinary and intercultural collaboration. She also thanks her family—Pat, Aaron, and Jordan Bray—whose encouragement and understanding have been invaluable. Her extended family deserves thanks, as well, for providing insights about the nature of culture and individual personality.

Laura expresses her personal thanks to Nadine Grimm, who was an invaluable source of much assistance and support while writing, and to Richard F. Rakos, for many productive conversations during the development and drafting of these ideas. She is also grateful to her ever-supportive husband W. Paul Meyer, for his calm encouragement and enthusiasm. Her greatest debt, however, is to her coauthors, for one of the best collaborative writing experiences of her scholarly life.

Andy thanks Bette and Laura for making the development of this text one of the most stimulating and intellectually rewarding projects of his career; that it also has been great fun is a testament to their talents and personalities. He also recognizes the tremendous support of Tina S. Miracle, his wife of more than three decades, who shouldered a considerable share of the responsibilities on another project so that he could devote more time and energy to this one.

ABOUT THE AUTHORS

Bette R. Bonder, PhD, OTR/L, FAOTA, Professor of Health Sciences and Psychology at Cleveland State University, is an occupational therapist and psychologist with experience working with individuals from diverse backgrounds in mental health, gerontology, and developmental disabilities. She is currently engaged in a study of the meaning of occupation for older adults, including examination of cultural factors that affect occupational choice and interpretation.

Laura Martin, PhD, Associate Dean of Arts and Sciences and Professor of Anthropology and Modern Languages at Cleveland State University, is a linguist with extensive fieldwork experience in the United States and Central American cultures, especially Mayan cultures. She has taught languages, linguistics, fieldwork methodologies, and a variety of cultural courses, and has conducted research on cultural issues in educational settings, including study-abroad settings and in health-related contexts.

Andrew W. Miracle, PhD, Associate Dean of Health and Urban Affairs and Professor of Public Health at Florida International University, is an anthropologist with fieldwork experience in South America and in educational settings in the United States, including studies on the effects of school sports on athletes and communities. He has published articles and books on human sexuality, including a forthcoming text coauthored with his wife, Tina S. Miracle, and Roy F. Baumeister.

PREFACE

This book presents a novel approach to the issue of cultural diversity in health care settings. It is in part a response to the repeated calls for greater use of interdisciplinary approaches in addressing the pressing concerns of health care professionals. Among these concerns, of course, is the increasing diversity among health professions, providers, patients, and institutions—each group marked by culture-based variation and each in constant contact with the others. Few topics lend themselves as well to interdisciplinary perspectives as the matter of cultural diversity because culture itself encompasses the full range of human behaviors, organizations, values, and patterns. This work can provide students and professionals with important insights and techniques for handling a variety of cultural factors in clinical settings, regardless of the setting, profession, or cultural background of the participants.

This work has evolved from our own diverse interdisciplinary training and experiences. Our backgrounds include formal training and teaching expertise in the fields of psychology, linguistics, anthropology, sociology, education, occupational therapy, and foreign language. Some of us have direct clinical and consulting experience; all of us have done field-based research using ethnographic methods, a cornerstone of the approach taken in this book. Our subject populations have included non-Western cultures in Central and South America and the United States. We have all supervised study-abroad programs and designed educational programs for, with, and about persons from other countries. Each of us has a history of collaborative research and writing and moves comfortably across a variety of institutional contexts and multicultural settings.

As we began to talk about the various observations made throughout this period of developing expertise, we discovered that we shared a deep concern about the way in which professionals are trained to deal with cultural diversity. We also realized that we had in common a methodological perspective grounded in an inquiry-based ethnographic method that we believed could be learned and taught. From that point, we were determined to produce a manual that would assist learners and teachers in developing the skills and mental outlook that makes this method work.

This book can be used by individuals and in groups, by students and by working professionals in disciplines from physical therapy to nursing and from medicine to social work, in a variety of contexts from workshops to courses, and in many settings, including hospitals, clinics, universities, and private study groups. Every effort has been made to include examples that reflect the diversity of the expected audiences. Ancillary materials that can expand the material of the book and assist in using it successfully have also been prepared.

The first of these additional resources is an instructor's manual that we consider essential for anyone using this book as a classroom text. The manual contains additional exercises, resource lists, study guides, materials for student assessment such as examination questions and topics, and duplicable handouts for classroom use. It is available to adoptors at the SLACK website: *http://www.efacultylounge.com*. We also have a website, which will continue to expand and is intended to include such items as updated web resource links, additional case studies and exercises, sample course syllabi and other classroom materials, notices of workshop opportunities, and, most importantly, opportunities for feedback and interaction with us and other readers and users. Our web address is *http://health.csuohio.edu/healthculture*.

As even a cursory scan of the book will show, the goal has been maximum interaction between reader and text. The emphasis on constant questioning (including self-critique) and thoughtful interaction with the examples and your colleagues is a reflection of the methodology presented in the text. In keeping with this philosophy, we are eager to interact with those who use the text. You are encouraged to write or e-mail us in care of SLACK with your own examples and with news of successful applications of the book in your experience. Suggestions for improvement and comments about the book are also invited. We hope to use the website as a mechanism for establishing an ongoing, productive dialogue with practitioners, students, teachers, and other colleagues around the issues raised here and the strategies offered for understanding and managing them in our professional work lives. Treat the book as a conversation—a conversation you have with your students, your clients, your supervisors, and your coworkers, as well as with us. We look forward to your reactions and reports.

CHAPTER

1

Introduction

CHAPTER OBJECTIVES

By the end of this chapter, the reader will be able to:

1. Discuss the reasons why cultural issues have become prominent in health care.
2. Describe typical definitions of culture and the factors they have in common.
3. Define and discuss the two main strategies for describing culture.
4. Describe typical approaches to defining cultural competence.
5. Describe the two main mechanisms typically employed to learn cultural competence.
6. Describe the differences between typical approaches and those used in this book.
7. List the strategies that will enhance learning while using this book.

Figure 1-1. Clinicians routinely encounter individuals from many cultures in their daily practice.

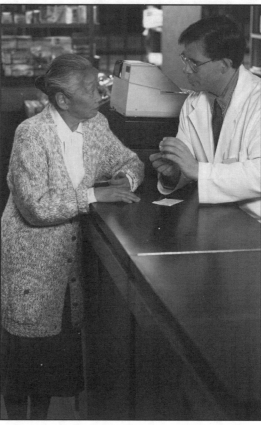

Culture. The term is everywhere around us. Culture contact. Culture shock. Culture conflict. All these terms and concepts are invoked to explain aspects of human behavior and human misunderstanding. Cultural diversity. Cultural tolerance. Cultural sensitivity. Cultural competence. These are concepts that suggest avenues for managing the encounters that involve persons of different cultural backgrounds. Even though we are surrounded by the terms and concepts, however, we are not always certain about how we should behave. We do not always understand how to put into practice the positive approaches to cultural difference or to recognize when they are needed. If our profession requires us to interact with a wide range of individuals—as health care practice does—we may be under special pressure to handle ourselves competently in **cross-cultural** situations (Figure 1-1).

Increasingly, health care practitioners are recognizing the importance of culture in their interactions with clients and colleagues. As the United States population becomes more diverse, practitioners face situations in which their clients' cultural backgrounds are clearly different from their own. Skills that enhance care providers' abilities to rec-

ognize different cultural values, beliefs, and practices and to incorporate such factors into intervention are likely to lead to more successful treatment outcomes. Professional groups are placing greater value on such skills not only because their client populations are more diverse but also because a more diverse group of individuals is joining the ranks of health care professions (C. H. Harris, 2000; Le Postallec, 1999; New Waves, 1993; Pruegger & Rogers, 1994; Sleek, 1998).

Educational standards for health care professionals routinely include cultural competence as a training requirement. For example, the American Occupational Therapy Association (AOTA) *Standards for Accreditation of an Occupational Therapy Educational Program* (AOTA, 1999) and the *Evaluative Criteria for Accreditation of Educational Programs for the Preparation of Physical Therapists* (Commission on Accreditation of Physical Therapy Education, 1998) both acknowledge the importance of **cultural sensitivity** for practitioner training. Some professions, among them the American Psychological Association (APA, 1990) and the American Medical Association (AMA, 1999), are attempting more specifically to identify the attributes of cultural competence. An array of conferences and continuing education programs across disciplines focus on cultural issues. For example, multiple sessions at the 2000 APA annual meeting and the 2000 annual conference of the American Speech and Hearing Association (ASHA) dealt with issues of cultural diversity. Because of increased emphasis on client-centered goals and intervention, culture has become a more central emphasis of treatment. "America is a country of many races and cultures, and with each passing year, more health care providers are recognizing the challenge of caring for patients from diverse linguistic and cultural backgrounds" (Fortier, 1999). Central to these efforts is the notion of culture itself.

Q 1-1. Before reading further, think about what the term culture means to you. Do you have in mind a formal definition of this core concept? Using the margins of this page, take a moment to list a few key terms that might be part of your definition of culture.

DEFINING CULTURE

Defining culture is notoriously difficult. Most scholars writing formal definitions of culture concur about some of its characteristics but still leave considerable ambiguity. A commonly cited characteristic of culture is that it is "shared by people." Also, culture is said to distinguish **insiders** from **outsiders**—those who are members of one cultural group from those who are not. Ambiguity results from what is left unspecified. What is the nature of "cultural groups"? How much experience, language, and values must members "share"? What if members share some but not all cultural knowledge with individuals "outside" the group, however that knowledge is defined? How much do you have to know before you are considered a "member" of the group? Attempts to circumscribe a single culture often do not account for the considerable variation that can exist in experiences, languages, values, or other traits that can coexist even within a clearly demarcated **society**. Even within relatively small groups of individuals, not everything is shared.

Q 1-2. Think for a moment about your own life. How would you respond to the question, "What cultural background do you come from?" What are the key features you use to decide what cultural identity to claim—particular religious traditions, ethnic heritage, family language, dress, or beliefs about what makes a good person? List some of these features at the end of the chapter. Would you say you are influenced by more than one cultural group or identity?

1-3. "Some Definitions of Culture" (see box on page 4) contains several formal definitions of culture in use among health care professional groups. Consider the similarities and differences among them.

1-4. Compare the boxed definitions to your own provisional definition developed earlier. What similarities and differences do you see among them? What concepts seem to be common to all the formal definitions? What do you think is missing from these definitions? How might the differences among the definitions lead to confusion in clinical settings?

DESCRIBING CULTURE

Found among these definitions are two general approaches to describing and understanding culture. These can be categorized as the descriptive approach and the rules approach. In this section, we will summarize both approaches, distinguishing them later from the approach taken in this book.

The Descriptive Approach

The **descriptive approach** to culture involves the systematic identification of the particular traits and material goods of a given society. A full description of all the technological, economic, political, kinship, and religious characteristics of a people, along with their socialization practices and value systems, has been assumed to provide a description of the culture of that people. Even though it is impossible to describe everything about a given people, providing a list of the major traits, patterns of behavior, and material objects produced or used can offer a good approximation of a particular culture at a given moment in time. This approach assumes that by describing what seem to be significant traits of a culture, outsiders can gain an appreciation of what life is like for the people involved. Producing such descriptions is a demanding task.

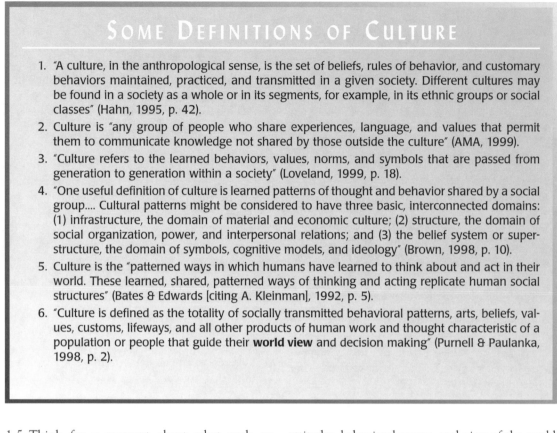

SOME DEFINITIONS OF CULTURE

1. "A culture, in the anthropological sense, is the set of beliefs, rules of behavior, and customary behaviors maintained, practiced, and transmitted in a given society. Different cultures may be found in a society as a whole or in its segments, for example, in its ethnic groups or social classes" (Hahn, 1995, p. 42).

2. Culture is "any group of people who share experiences, language, and values that permit them to communicate knowledge not shared by those outside the culture" (AMA, 1999).

3. "Culture refers to the learned behaviors, values, norms, and symbols that are passed from generation to generation within a society" (Loveland, 1999, p. 18).

4. "One useful definition of culture is learned patterns of thought and behavior shared by a social group.... Cultural patterns might be considered to have three basic, interconnected domains: (1) infrastructure, the domain of material and economic culture; (2) structure, the domain of social organization, power, and interpersonal relations; and (3) the belief system or super-structure, the domain of symbols, cognitive models, and ideology" (Brown, 1998, p. 10).

5. Culture is the "patterned ways in which humans have learned to think about and act in their world. These learned, shared, patterned ways of thinking and acting replicate human social structures" (Bates & Edwards [citing A. Kleinman], 1992, p. 5).

6. "Culture is defined as the totality of socially transmitted behavioral patterns, arts, beliefs, values, customs, lifeways, and all other products of human work and thought characteristic of a population or people that guide their **world view** and decision making" (Purnell & Paulanka, 1998, p. 2).

Q 1-5. Think for a moment about what such an approach would require. Imagine you were asked to describe your own culture by making a list of all the foods associated with significant holidays or all the paraphernalia used at formal weddings. Choose one of these lists and spend 5 minutes writing down items that would appear on it. How far can you get? How long would it take to complete such a list? Did any questions occur to you about how to determine what goes on the list? What would a reader of your list learn about your culture?

Often cultures are summarized by just a few key values or characteristics. Such summaries, although useful (and some of which you will see in this book), are superficial and inadequate for real understanding of a cultural group. For example, there is a familiar cultural group we will refer to throughout this book as the "Old Americans" (Nayak, Shiflett, Eshun, & Levine, 2000). This term has nothing to do with age; rather, it refers to people who are descendants of individuals of European ancestry who were early settlers in the United States and whose culture is often considered the "majority" culture in the country. It is the group whose values, attitudes, behavioral norms, and view of the world generally dominate in American society, including in health care institutions. This is the group whose values and behaviors dominate media representations of the United States.

We might summarize this culture as having a capitalist economic system, Protestant religious foundation, and a strong emphasis on individualism and hard work. Eating habits of the group include consumption of fast food, white bread, red meat, and soda. Culturally important holidays include major Christian festivals, especially Christmas, and national holidays such as Thanksgiving and Independence Day. Such a summary, while providing some information, hardly provides a useful description of contemporary American society. However, such summaries based largely on descriptive approaches to cultural interpretation, are often all we know about less familiar cultures.

1-6. Consider your earlier list of food or wedding paraphernalia. Does it generally reflect an Old American cultural background or some other ethnic or cultural group? If it does represent an Old American tradition, how well does your list relate to our summary of that group? **Q**

The Rules Approach

The **rules approach** to describing culture assumes that culture is a cognitive model of reality rather than a list of goods or behaviors. Thus, understanding a culture means knowing how a people view reality, how they make distinctions among categories of things, and how they generally make decisions about right courses of action. Taking a rules approach to Old American culture, one would explain the rules of behavior that direct social behavior such as the ones that organize use of personal space or determine whom one can touch under what circumstances. Of course, in taking this approach it is necessary to know (and to describe for others) most of the things that exist in the world of those people. In this sense, the rules approach subsumes the descriptive one. Not everything can be included in a rules study, nor can it ever be known with certainty that the model provided by such an approach really describes the culture held by all the people in a society or even that of most of them.

Q

1-7. To get a sense of how a rules approach to cultural description works, consider the rules used by Old Americans for dealing with childbirth, for preparing for Thanksgiving, or for greeting strangers. Spend 5 minutes formulating two or three rules in one of these categories.

1-8. What did you need to know to develop such rules? What do you need to describe in order for the rules to make sense to someone of another cultural background? Does your own cultural background lead you to feel like an insider or an outsider when compared with Old American culture?

Old American culture may be among the most familiar or most widely recognized in the United States. However, like most societies ours has a mixture of cultural traditions. The United States can be thought of as a complex society, because the mixture of traditions is great. There is variation in all cultural groups, no matter how small; but in complex societies this variation is extensive, as it is in the United States. As we have seen, definitions of culture also vary, often according to the purposes they serve. In this book, we develop a definition of culture with pragmatic meaning for health care practitioners. In our definition, which we discuss in detail later, we emphasize the ways in which the combination of experience, environment, and personal preference results in each individual having a unique set of cultural patterns. Although our definition is more complex than the simple descriptive and rules approaches suggest, it is also more appropriate and adaptable to the special demands of **intercultural** interaction in health care settings.

DEFINING CULTURAL COMPETENCE

Like culture, **cultural competence** is a difficult concept to define. What do you have to know to be culturally competent? What do you have to do? How can you know when cross-cultural encounters are successful? There is considerable controversy over whether cultural competency activities are worthwhile at all (*Physician's Weekly*, 2000). Some individuals feel that cultural competency improves the quality of clinical care; others perceive the term as having become a euphemism for a kind of political correctness. The controversy may reflect the fact that, as with culture, there are multiple definitions of cultural competence and lists of the skills required to achieve it. Often, such lists present an ambitious and perhaps unrealistic set of expectations about a health care provider's ability and resources for dealing with cultural complexity or diversity.

1-9. Consider the APA (1993) guidelines for providing culturally appropriate care (see box on pages 6-7). Do you think they are complete?

Q

1-10. In each numbered item in the APA guidelines, a series of resources is implied or assumed. For example, item 1 assumes availability of the relevant written material in whatever language a client understands. Choose two guidelines and make a list of the resources each assumes.

1-11. Each numbered guideline also makes **assumptions** about the abilities and aptitudes of the client and therapist. For example, item 1 assumes the client's language has a written form and that the client is literate in it. Choose two guidelines and make notes about the assumptions expressed about the two participants.

1-12. Consider item 9, which identifies a series of cultural factors assumed to be "relevant." Can you think of factors that should be added? Are

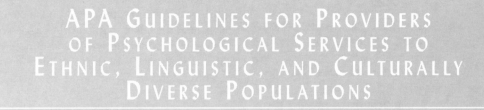

APA Guidelines for Providers of Psychological Services to Ethnic, Linguistic, and Culturally Diverse Populations

Preamble: The Guidelines represent general principles that are intended to be aspirational in nature and are designed to provide suggestions to psychologists in working with ethnically, linguistically, and culturally diverse populations.

1. Psychologists educate their clients to the process of psychological intervention, such as goals and expectations; the scope and, where appropriate, legal limit of confidentiality; and the psychologists' orientations.

   a. Whenever possible, psychologists provide information in writing along with oral explanations.

   b. Whenever possible, the written information is provided in the language understandable to the client.

2. Psychologists are cognizant of relevant research and practice issues as related to the population being served.

   a. Psychologists acknowledge that ethnicity and culture impact on behavior and take those factors into account when working with various ethnic/racial groups.

   b. Psychologists seek out education and training experiences to enhance their understanding to address the needs of these populations more appropriately and effectively. These experiences include cultural, social, psychological, political, economic, and historical material specific to the particular ethnic group being served.

   c. Psychologists recognize the limits of their competencies and expertise. Psychologists who do not possess knowledge and training about an ethnic group seek consultation with, and/or make referrals to, appropriate experts as necessary.

   d. Psychologists consider the validity of given instruments or procedures and interpret resulting data, keeping in mind the cultural and linguistic characteristics of the person being assessed. Psychologists are aware of the test's reference population and possible limitations of such instruments with other populations.

3. Psychologists recognize ethnicity and culture as significant parameters in understanding psychological processes.

   a. Psychologists, regardless of ethnic or racial background, are aware of how their own cultural background, experiences, attitudes, values, and biases influence psychological processes. They make efforts to correct any prejudices and biases.

   b. Psychologists' practice incorporates an understanding of the client's ethnic and cultural background. This includes the client's familiarity and comfort with the majority culture as well as ways in which the client's culture may add to or improve various aspects of the majority culture and/or of society at large.

   c. Psychologists help clients increase their awareness of their own cultural values and norms, and they facilitate discovery of ways clients can apply this awareness to their own lives and to society at large.

   d. Psychologists seek to help a client determine whether a "problem" stems from racism or bias in others so that the client does not inappropriately personalize problems.

   e. Psychologists consider not only differential diagnostic issues but also cultural beliefs and values of the clients and his/her community in providing intervention.

4. Psychologists respect the roles of family members and community structures, hierarchies, values, and beliefs within the client's culture.

   a. Psychologists identify resources in the family and the larger community.

   b. Clarification of the role of the psychologist and the expectations of the client precede

continued

intervention. Psychologists seek to ensure that both the psychologist and client have a clear understanding of what services and roles are reasonable.

5. Psychologists respect clients' religious and/or spiritual beliefs and values, including attributions and taboos, since they affect world view, psychosocial functioning, and expressions of distress.

   a. Part of working in minority communities is to become familiar with indigenous beliefs and practices and to respect them.

   b. Effective psychological intervention may be aided by consultation with and/or inclusion of religious and spiritual leaders or practitioners relevant to the client's culture and belief systems.

6. Psychologists interact in the language requested by the client and, if this is not feasible, make an appropriate referral.

   a. Problems may arise when the linguistic skills of the psychologist do not match the language of the client. In such a case, psychologists refer the client to a mental health professional who is competent to interact in the language of the client. If this is not possible, psychologists offer the client a translator with cultural knowledge and an appropriate professional background. When no translator is available, then a trained paraprofessional from the client's culture is used as a translator or culture broker.

   b. If translation is necessary, psychologists do not retain the services of translators or paraprofessionals who may have dual roles with the client to avoid jeopardizing the validity of evaluation or the effectiveness of intervention.

   c. Psychologists interpret and relate the test data in terms understandable and relevant to the needs of those assessed.

7. Psychologists consider the impact of adverse social, environmental, and political factors in assessing problems and designing interventions.

   a. Types of intervention strategies to be used match to the client's level of need (e.g., Maslow's hierarchy of needs).

   b. Psychologists work within the cultural setting to improve the welfare of all persons concerned, if there is a conflict between cultural values and human rights.

8. Psychologists attend to as well as work to eliminate biases, prejudices, and discriminatory practices.

   a. Psychologists acknowledge relevant discriminatory practices at the social and community level may be affecting the psychological welfare of the population being served.

   b. Psychologists are cognizant of sociopolitical contexts in conducting evaluations and providing interventions; they develop sensitivity to issues of oppression, sexism, elitism, and racism.

9. Psychologists working with culturally diverse populations should document culturally and sociopolitically relevant factors in the records.

   a. Number of generations in the country

   b. Number of years in the country

   c. Fluency in English

   d. Extent of family support (or disintegration of family)

   e. Community resources

   f. Level of education

   g. Change in social status as a result of coming to this country (for immigrant or refugee)

   h. Intimate relationships with people of different backgrounds

   i. Level of stress related to acculturation

there some factors listed that might not be relevant? Overall, what cultural assumptions by the profession seem to underlie the listed factors?

Q 1-13. What methods can you think of to evaluate how well a therapist meets these standards?

Some persons might dispute that the goals set out by the APA are realistic or appropriate. Even those who believe this list is reflective of genuine cultural competence might have difficulty evaluating a practitioner's success at accomplishing these actions. Other factors exist in health care settings that affect achievement of such goals.

STRATEGIES FOR BECOMING CULTURALLY COMPETENT

In clinical settings, efforts to recognize and respect culture are complicated by organizational and practical considerations. There are cost pressures to minimize time spent with each individual and to focus on preselected intervention goals that reflect organizational rather than personal goals. Cultural competence in such settings requires both individual and organizational efforts (Ramos, 2000). Still, the recognition that cultural factors play an important role in health outcomes compels practitioners and their organizations to tackle the complexities of culturally sensitive care.

To address these complexities, two main types of approaches have been employed: what we might call **fact-centered** and **attitude-centered** approaches. The fact-centered training approach is widely used by consultants to health care organizations.

A common method of teaching cultural competence is to provide a general overview of the role of culture in health service delivery and then to spend time focusing on the health beliefs and behaviors of specific ethnic groups. While this has the effect of increasing general knowledge about an ethnic population, it can lead to facile stereotyping. (DiversityRx, 1997a)

In a fact-centered approach, individuals strive to learn about particular cultures. What do African-Americans believe about health and illness? How do Hispanic families interact? What are the beliefs of Asians about interpersonal relationships? The advantage of such an approach is that it provides the clinician with a starting place for interacting with a particular individual. Some amount of factual knowledge is vital to effective cross-cultural interaction and it is possible to design programming to focus on a single group (DiversityRx, 1997a).

However, there are a number of weaknesses inherent in a fact-centered approach to culture. First, it is impossible to know all there is to know about every culture. After all, African-American, Hispanic, and Asian are not single cultures, but many. The category "African-American" can include second-generation Afro-Cubans as well as descendants from Philadelphia's pre-Civil War free Black community. "Hispanic" may encompass both recent immigrants from El Salvador and individuals whose families have been living for some 500 years in what is now New Mexico. Hmong immigrants who came to the United States at the end of the Vietnam War and Chinese-Americans whose ancestors arrived in San Francisco in the 19th century may both be considered "Asian."

Moreover, each culture changes over time, and it is important to know not just the attributes of a culture at a particular point, but also the historical influences that have affected its development. Wars, displacement, and new technologies, among many other factors, all affect the ways in which particular cultures develop. Without knowledge and information about such influences, it is possible to develop stereotypical views of cultures that may be somewhat pejorative. Furthermore, even if one could learn all there is to know about, say, Vietnamese culture, the individual you are treating is not only Vietnamese, but has other important experiences that influence health and health care. For example, he or she is first, second, or third generation; lives in an urban, suburban, or rural setting; and has a professional or blue-collar occupation. Any individual inevitably has multiple social influences on her or his health-related behaviors. In addition, individual personality serves as a lens through which specific cultural information is viewed. A person is not a collection of cultural "facts" but rather a complex bundle of cultural influences and other factors that impact perceptions and sentiments as well as behaviors.

Finally, a fact-centered approach risks replacing one stereotype with another. The new stereotype may be more positive but still fail to capture the complex nature of culture. "While information about specific cultures can contribute to understanding, superficial knowledge sometimes leads to stereotyping that belies the complexity of cultural issues and the nature of the individual" (DiversityRx, 1997a).

A second approach to training in cultural sensitivity is attitude-centered. This approach emphasizes the importance of valuing all cultures. Practitioners seek to examine their own beliefs, and to recognize and avoid negative stereotypes and perceptions. The obvious advantage of such an approach is its acknowledgment of the centrality of culture and its encouragement of positive attitudes. Research, however, is equivocal about whether educational programs can actually alter attitudes to any significant extent (Pruegger & Rogers, 1994). Furthermore, positive attitude does not necessarily lead to behavior change, nor does it provide one with the tools to behave in an effective manner. Good intentions are not enough to ensure competent interaction across cultural boundaries. What is needed is a new approach to culture that enables practitioners to gather and use needed information in framing interventions.

OUR APPROACH TO CULTURE AND CULTURAL COMPETENCE

This book takes a third approach to culture and cultural competence. Our goal is to offer a definition of culture and an approach to cultural competence that afford a practical guide to effective interaction in clinical and professional settings by providing specific tools and knowledge. The first novel aspect of our philosophy lies in our definition of culture. We view culture as constantly emergent. In the term **culture emergent** we emphasize the dynamic, nuanced, and contextual nature of culture, not its artifacts or rules. We recognize that culture is expressed through individual behavior reflective of the multiple influences that shape human experience. These expressions of cultural influences are always responsive to immediate context. Culture emerges in interactions among individuals, primarily through talk, and is conditioned by transient circumstances as well as by traditional patterns of behavior. Rather than attempt to define and delineate specific cultural groups, we take the approach that the way any individual behaves is based on the array of influences unique to her or his development. In complex societies, most individuals are in contact with multiple cultural influences and different contexts elicit different behaviors.

Our method is also novel as applied to cultural competence. We introduce an **inquiry-centered approach** to cultural competence (Johnson, Hardt, & Kleinman, 1995). This approach is drawn from the long history of anthropology and other disciplines that focus on "learning how to ask" (Bohannon & Van der Eist, 1998; Briggs, 1986). It is most closely associated with **ethnography** and "field-based" research. Ethnographic methodology reflects a particular mindset and offers a practical and learnable strategy for interacting with individuals to elicit cultural information critical to good care. This methodology allows us to provide a specific set of tools and skills for effective clinical interactions in intercultural settings, without regard to which particular culture is represented by the patient.

Sue (2000) defines three important characteristics that providers need in order to engage in effective intercultural intervention. This book presents a strategy for helping providers acquire them.

- **Scientific-mindedness**. Culturally effective providers form hypotheses before information gathering rather than draw conclusions about cultural issues. They develop creative ways to test their hypotheses and then act on the basis of acquired data. It is important to remember that hypotheses are built on prior observation and experience. They may be discarded or supported; the scientist tests initial guesses and acts based on systematically acquired data.

- **Dynamic sizing skills**. Culturally effective providers recognize situations in which to generalize or individualize when interacting with clients. "Facts" about a cultural group help in generating hypotheses. Comparison of data about the individual with those facts lets the clinician decide whether they fit the specific situation.

- **Culture-specific expertise**. Culturally effective providers know and understand their clients' cultural groups, the environments in which they live, and intervention techniques useful to working with such clients. This baseline information is a foundation from which evidence can be assessed about the individual and his or her similarities and differences when compared with culture-specific information. In every situation there is an interplay between the general and the individual.

Finally, because it is becoming essential to evaluate whether practitioners are providing culturally relevant care, we also present a set of assessment and intervention strategies that can increase effective response to cultural factors in clinical interaction (Spencer, Krefting, & Mattingly, 1993).

USING THIS BOOK

In our experience, acknowledging the importance of culture and placing value on cultural competence do not always translate into overt behavior. We have already seen that one reason may be that terms and goals are not clear. Defining culture is sufficiently difficult that social scientists have argued for years without arriving at a single consensus definition. Culture is complex and changes over time. Individuals experience multiple cultural influences during the course of their lives. A great deal of research focuses on ethnic or racial identity, assuming that an individual fits only one group; in reality, everyone belongs to a multitude of cultural groups (Hong, Morris, Chiu, & Benet-Martinez, 2000).

Other factors, however, relate to the difficulty in finding specific actions to perform to ensure cultural competence. It is hard work to adopt the perspective of another or to discover information deemed necessary for appropriate action. Covert conflicts in values or our fears of cultural difference may inhibit our ability to adopt a culturally sensitive mindset or to adjust our own behaviors in order to accommodate the behavioral norms of others.

With this book, we propose to remedy some of these difficulties in specific ways: with clear writing and definitions, with numerous examples and opportunities to think through the relevance and implications of terms, with detailed suggestions for action in your own practice, with exercises to help you build the skills required, and with direct efforts to deal with the covert elements that subvert culturally effective practice. We adopt the view that the factors that create culturally attentive practice will enhance all clinical encounters, as all of us—practitioners and patients alike—are complex bundles of cultural traits, as well as unique personalities.

This book provides you with the tools you need to engage in effective intercultural interactions regardless of your own culture and that of the client. These tools are useful every time you provide care, not just when the other person seems obviously different from you. In the first few chapters we develop our theory and lay the groundwork for our methodology. We begin in Chapter 2 by expanding our definition of culture emergent and giving a description of the components of culture that are important to health care providers. In Chapter 3, we consider the interaction of biological, environmental, and personal characteristics with cultural influences. In Chapter 4, we examine the specific impact of culture on health beliefs and practices.

The next two chapters deal directly with methods and skills development. In Chapter 5 we discuss issues involved in observing and evaluating individual cultural influences, followed in Chapter 6 by a description of specific ways to negotiate cultural differences with clients and coworkers. The final chapters relate specifically to health care practice. Chapter 7 is a discussion of mechanisms that can elicit individual cultural beliefs and incorporate them effectively into clinical practice. Finally, in Chapter 8 we address mechanisms that enable practitioners to evaluate the success of their interventions and ensure that they have provided ethically and culturally sensitive treatment. Throughout the book, there are opportunities for readers to explore their own beliefs, examine case examples, and practice new skills.

Clinicians know that personal growth and increasing professional effectiveness require reflection and continual evaluation of outcomes. In addition, effective use of resources can enhance outcomes. Thus, we include opportunities for self-reflection and consideration of an array of typical clinical situations, as well as reference materials for further exploration. You will find a variety of different kinds of examples that introduce you to a number of different cultures, some of which you may feel you know well; others will be new to you. Some are brief examples intended to illustrate particular points raised in the text. Some of the examples are extended case studies, presented with more detailed cultural information. Some examples are like threads woven through the text, reappearing to provide additional information as you read more. Each chapter opens with a boxed excerpt from an extended case study. This unfolding case clarifies and crystallizes the potential for cultural conflict among caring and well-intended individuals, and encourages reflection on alternative strategies for interaction. All these examples are designed to reproduce the experience of learning about culture as it actually happens, that is, through the gradual revelations that occur in real encounters.

There are also a series of other boxes throughout the book. Some boxes present questions and exercises designed to help you process the information contained in the text; others provide additional examples or supplemental reference materials. As you read the examples, it will be helpful to reflect on your reactions to them. Do they make sense to you? Do they generate an emotional response? What kind of response? Many of our personal reactions are the result of our own cultural values and beliefs. For example, in reading the term Old American, one individual—a gerontologist—perceived a slight against elders, even though our definition has no relationship to age. Recall that we use the term to label "mainstream" American culture—that of families that have been in the United States for many generations. As you will read in Chapter 5, the reader's response is an example of vantage, the unavoidable reaction of individuals as they process and perceive events from their own unique perspective. Every reaction provides an opportunity for reflection about your vantage.

The best use of this book requires you to be a responsive reader. As you read, you will want to spend some time reflecting on the examples and exercises. Consider not only what they tell you about specific cases and cultures, but also what they tell you of learning about culture. Whenever you are asked to pause and reflect, or to make notes and respond to questions, take time to do so. Space is provided at the end of each chapter for you to make notes and respond to exercises.

Effective cultural interaction requires a mindset that is open to surprise and reflection and allows you to make connections. You will find that the structure of the book is much like that of clinical encounters. Not all the information is presented immediately. Try to read with the active curiosity that facilitates cultural interaction. In clinical encounters, you can never acquire all the knowledge you will need about your clients' cultures, but you can acquire the skills and mindset that facilitate your comfort and effectiveness. You should treat this book as a kind of workbook or journal. It invites your direct interaction. As you gather new information, your perceptions will undoubtedly change.

This gradual unfolding is typical of all human interaction; there is always more to learn, even about your closest friend.

Q

1-14. Take a moment now to reflect on the term Old American. What did you think the term meant when you first read it? How do you feel about it as a description of mainstream American culture? Is there a term you think would be better?

We encourage you to keep a journal as you read this book. In your journal you can include your personal reactions to what you learn, your reflections on your own values and behaviors, and questions raised by the material. We also suggest that you record observations from your daily life as you learn more about intercultural interaction. We provide space at the end of chapters for you to do this kind of journaling. A journal provides an outlet for your thoughts as you read and a way to examine changes in your understanding over time.

Clinicians must ask their clients for help in understanding the value systems from which they come. And they should make sure their clients feel that any cultural differences they may have with the clinician are respected and acknowledged during the therapy process. (Sleek, 1998)

Although this goal seems obvious, enacting this set of beliefs is complex, requiring a set of specific strategies on the part of practitioners. This book provides those strategies, as well as practice in their enactment and evaluation of these behaviors. We invite you to proceed now toward your own goal of improving your cross-cultural awareness and skills.

MINI-ETHNOGRAPHY

Introduction

Although now somewhat dated, the following ethnography-based article (Miner, 1956) provides insight into the activities of a magic-ridden society and poses questions about the nature of culture, ritual, and health. The article is also valuable in illustrating the utility of the **ethnographic approach**. Stepping outside of the familiar and describing the activities of a particular people can be extremely useful. The article provides an eye-opening view of activities that otherwise might be assumed to be so commonplace as to be value-free. Further, the article challenges our belief systems by presenting a new perspective on this particular group. Durante describes a perspective proposed by Melford Spiro, "(T)here exists in ethnography a certain playful element which consists of changing the similar into the strange and, vice versa, the strange into the familiar" (Durante, 1997, p. 86).

continued

Body Ritual Among the Nacirema, by Horace Miner

Miner, H. (1956). Body ritual among the Nacirema. *American Anthropologist, 58,* 503-507.
Reprinted with permission.

The anthropologist has become so familiar with the diversity of ways in which different peoples behave in similar situations that he is not apt to be surprised by even the most exotic customs. In fact, if all of the logically possible combinations of behavior have not been found somewhere in the world, he is apt to suspect that they must be present in some yet undescribed tribe. This point has, in fact, been expressed by Murdock (1949:71) with respect to clan organization. In this light, the magical beliefs and practices of the Nacirema present such unusual aspects that it seems desirable to describe them as an example of the extremes to which human behavior can go.

Professor Linton first brought the ritual of the Nacirema to the attention of anthropologists 20 years ago (1936:326), but the culture of this people is still very poorly understood. They are a North American group living in the territory between the Canadian Cree, the Yaqui and Tarahumara of Mexico, and the Carib and Arawak of the Antilles. Little is known of their origin, although tradition states that they came from the east. According to Nacirema mythology, their nation was originated by a culture hero, Notgnihsaw, who is otherwise known for two great feats of strength—the throwing of a piece of wampum across the river Pa-To-Mac and the chopping down of a cherry tree in which the Spirit of Truth resided.

Nacirema culture is characterized by a highly developed market economy which has evolved in a rich natural habit. While much of the people's time is devoted to economic pursuits, a large part of the fruits of these labors and a considerable portion of the day are spent in ritual activity. The focus of this activity is the human body, the appearance and health of which loom as a dominant concern in the ethos of the people. While such a concern is certainly not unusual, its ceremonial aspects and associated philosophy are unique.

The fundamental belief underlying the whole system appears to be that the human body is ugly and that its natural tendency is to debility and disease. Incarcerated in such a body, man's only hope is to avert these characteristics through the use of the powerful influences of ritual and ceremony. Every household has one or more shrines devoted to this purpose. The more powerful individuals in the society have several shrines in their houses and, in fact, the opulence of a house is often referred to in terms of the number of such ritual centers it possesses. Most houses are wattle and daub construction, but the shrine rooms of the more wealthy are walled with stone. Poorer families imitate the rich by applying pottery plaques to their shrine walls.

While each family has at least one such shrine, the rituals associated with it are not family ceremonies but are private and secret. The rites are normally only discussed with children, and then only during the period when they are being initiated into these mysteries. I was able, however, to establish sufficient rapport with the natives to examine these shrines and to have the rituals described to me.

The focal point of the shrine is a box or chest which is built into the wall. In this chest are kept the many charms and magical potions without which no native believes he could live. These preparations are secured from a variety of specialized practitioners. The most powerful of these are the medicine men, whose assistance must be rewarded with substantial gifts. However, the medicine men do not provide the curative potions for their clients, but decide what the ingredients should be and then write them down in an ancient and secret language. This writing is understood only by the medicine men and by the herbalists who, for another gift, provide the required charm.

The charm is not disposed of after it has served its purpose, but is placed in the charm-box of the household shrine. As the magical materials are specific for certain ills, and the real or imagined maladies of the people are many, the charm-box is usually full to overflowing. The magical packets are so numerous that people forget what their purposes were and fear to use them again. While the natives are very vague on this point, we can only assume that the idea in retaining all the old magical materials is that their presence in the charm-box, before which the body rituals are conducted, will in some way protect the worshipper.

Beneath the charm-box is a small font. Each day every member of the family, in succession, enters the shrine room, bows his head before the charm-box, mingles different sorts of holy water in the font, and proceeds with a brief rite of ablution. The holy waters are secured from the

continued

Water Temple of the community, where the priests conduct elaborate ceremonies to make the liquid ritually pure.

In the hierarchy of magical practitioners, and below the medicine men in the prestige, are specialists whose designation is best translated "holy-mouth-men." The Nacirema have an almost pathological horror of and fascination with the mouth, the condition of which is believed to have supernatural influence on all social relationships. Were it not for the rituals of the mouth, they believe that their teeth would fall out, their gums bleed, their jaws shrink, their friends desert them, and their lovers reject them. (They also believe that a strong relationship exists between oral and moral characteristics. For example, there is a ritual ablution of the mouth for children which is supposed to improve their moral fiber.)

The daily body ritual performed by everyone includes a mouth-rite. Despite the fact that these people are so punctilious about care of the mouth, this rite involves a practice which strikes the uninitiated stranger as revolting. It was reported to me that the ritual consists of inserting a small bundle of hog hairs in the mouth, along with certain magical powders, and then moving the bundle in a highly formalized series of gestures.

In addition to the private mouth-rite, the people seek out a holy-mouth-man once or twice a year. These practitioners have an impressive set of paraphernalia, consisting of a variety of augers, awls, probes, and prods. The use of these objects in the exorcism of the evils of the mouth involves almost unbelievable ritual torture of the client. The holy-mouth-man opens the client's mouth, and using the above mentioned tools, enlarges any holes which decay may have created in the teeth. Magical materials are put into these holes. If there are no naturally occurring holes in the teeth, large sections of one or more teeth are gouged out so that the supernatural substance can be applied. In the client's view, the purpose of these ministrations is to arrest decay and to draw friends. The extremely sacred and traditional character of the rite is evident in the fact that the natives return to the holy-mouth-men year after year, despite the fact that their teeth continue to decay.

It is hoped that, when a thorough study of the Nacirema is made, there will be careful inquiry into the personality structure of these people. One has but to watch the gleam in the eye of a holy-mouth-man as he jabs an awl into an exposed nerve to suspect that a certain amount of sadism is involved. If this can be established, a very interesting pattern emerges, for most of the population shows definite masochistic tendencies. It was to these that Professor Linton referred in discussing a distinctive part of the daily body ritual which is performed only by men. This part of the rite involves scraping and lacerating the surface of the face with a sharp instrument. Special women's rites are performed only four times during each lunar month, but what they lack in frequency is made up in barbarity. As part of this ceremony, women bake their heads in small ovens for about an hour. The theoretically interesting point is that what seems to be preponderantly masochistic people have developed sadistic specialists.

The medicine men have an imposing temples or *latipso*, in every community of any size. The more elaborate ceremonies required to treat very sick patients can only be performed at this temple. These ceremonies involve not only the thaumaturge but a permanent group of vestal maidens who move sedately about the temple chambers in distinctive costume and headdress.

The *latipso* ceremonies are so harsh that it is phenomenal that a fair proportion of the really sick natives who enter the temple ever recover. Small children whose indoctrination is still incomplete have been known to resist attempts to take them to the temple because "that is where you go to die." Despite this fact, sick adults are not only willing, but eager to undergo the protracted ritual purification, if they can afford to do so. No matter how ill the supplicant or how grave the emergency, the guardians of many temples will not admit a client if he cannot give a rich gift to the custodian. Even after one has gained admission and survived the ceremonies, the guardians will not permit the neophyte to leave until he makes still another gift.

The supplicant entering the temple is first stripped of all his or her clothes. In everyday life the Nacirema avoids exposure of his body and its natural functions. Bathing and excretory acts are performed only in the secrecy of the household shrine, where they are ritualized as part of the body-rites. Psychological shock results from the fact that body secrecy is suddenly lost upon entry into the *latipso*. A man, whose own wife has never seen him in an excretory act, suddenly finds him-

continued

self naked and assisted by a vestal maiden while he performs his natural functions into a sacred vessel. This sort of ceremonial treatment is necessitated by the fact that the excreta are used by a diviner to ascertain the course and nature of the client's sickness. Female clients, on the other hand, find their naked bodies are subjected to the scrutiny, manipulation, and prodding of the medicine men.

Few supplicants in the temple are well enough to do anything but lie on their hard beds. The daily ceremonies, like the rites of the holy-mouth-men, involve discomfort and torture. With ritual precision, the vestals awaken their miserable charges each dawn and roll them about on their beds of pain while performing ablutions, in the formal movements of which the maidens are highly trained. At other times they insert magic wands in the supplicant's mouth or force him to eat substances which are supposed to be healing. From time to time the medicine men come to their clients and jab magically treated needles into their flesh. The fact that these temple ceremonies may not cure, and may even kill the neophyte, in no way decreases the people's faith in the medicine men.

There remains one other kind of practitioner, known as a "listener." This witch-doctor has the power to exorcise the devils that lodge in the heads of people who have been bewitched. The Nacirema believe that parents bewitch their own children. Mothers are particularly suspected of putting a curse on children while teaching them the secret body rituals. The counter-magic of the witch-doctor is unusual in its lack of ritual. The patient simply tells the "listener" all his troubles and fears, beginning with the earliest difficulties he can remember. The memory displayed by the Nacirema in these exorcism sessions is truly remarkable. It is not uncommon for the patient to bemoan the rejection he felt upon being weaned as a babe, and a few individuals even see their troubles going back to the traumatic effects of their own birth.

In conclusion, mention must be made of certain practices which have their base in native esthetics but which depend upon the pervasive aversion to the natural body and its functions. There are ritual fasts to make fat people thin and ceremonial feasts to make thin people fat. Still other rites are used to make women's breasts large if they are small, and smaller if they are large. General dissatisfaction with breast shape is symbolized in the fact that the ideal form is virtually outside the range of human variation. A few women afflicted with almost inhuman hyper-mammary development are so idolized that they make a handsome living by simply going from village to village and permitting the natives to stare at them for a fee.

Reference has already been made to the fact that excretory functions are ritualized, routinized, and relegated to secrecy. Natural reproductive functions are similarly distorted. Intercourse is taboo as a topic and scheduled as an act. Efforts are made to avoid pregnancy by the use of magical materials or by limiting intercourse to certain phases of the moon. Conception is actually very infrequent. When pregnant, women dress so as to hide their condition. Parturition takes place in secret, without friends or relatives to assist, and the majority of women do not nurse their infants.

Our review of the ritual life of the Nacirema has certainly shown them to be a magic-ridden people. It is hard to understand how they have managed to exist so long under the burdens which they have imposed upon themselves. But even such exotic customs as these take on real meaning when they are viewed with the insight provided by Malinowski when he wrote (1948:70):

Looking from far and above, from our high places of safety in the developed civilization, it is easy to see all the crudity and irrelevance of magic. But without its power and guidance early man could not have mastered his practical difficulties as he has done, nor could man have advanced to the higher stages of civilization.

References

Linton, R. (1936). *The Study of Man*. New York: Appleton-Century Co.

Malinowski, B. (1948). *Magic, Science, and Religion*. Glencoe: The Free Press.

Murdock, G. P. (1949). *Social Structure*. New York: The Macmillan Co.

continued

Considering the Mini-Ethnography

1-15. Miner writes in a style that mimics some of the features of traditional ethnographies, which put emphasis on cultural difference and exoticism. In some ways, it is a parody. At what point in the article did you first identify the cultural group being described?

1-16. If you are uncertain about the first question, reconsider the cultural group's name. It may help to read the name backwards (if you only now realize the identity of the group, read the article again before proceeding). How did you feel when you first identified the group?

1-17. How did you react to reading such routine acts as tooth-brushing described as a "mouth-rite" involving "bundles of hog hairs" and accompanied by "formalized… gestures"?

1-18. Were you able to detach yourself from the customary meanings of tooth-brushing and visits to the dentist ("holy-mouth-man") in order to imagine how these acts might be described as rituals or as magical, sacred events?

1-19. Reread the description of the *latipso* temple, ceremonies, and inhabitants ("guardians, vestal maidens, medicine men"). Think of the type of place where you practice (or will practice). Imagine that you are a first-time observer, from a completely different background. How might the organization, personnel, and activities of such a place be described by such an outsider?

1-20. Recall that many clients or patients may themselves be first-time observers and true outsiders when seeking your help. Choose one aspect of a health care practice site that is familiar to you and describe it as if you were new to it and seeing it for the first time.

1-21. One of the most valuable effects of a cultural description can be the way it makes us consider familiar cultural behaviors in a new light. Did Miner's essay give you a new perspective on health practice in the United States?

1-22. If you are not a native of the United States or if you have strong cultural influences from other traditions, reflect on your first experiences of toothpaste commercials, bathrooms, or health care settings. Does Miner's essay remind you of any of your own early reactions?

1-23. If you are using this book with a group, share your reactions to these questions with other group members and compare notes.

✎ NOTES ✐

Understanding Culture

CHAPTER OBJECTIVES

By the end of this chapter, the reader will be able to:

1. Define culture emergent.
2. Explain the processes by which culture is learned.
3. Distinguish between culture and society.
4. Discuss the importance of status positions and social roles.
5. Describe social roles as related to culture emergent.
6. Define and discuss role conflict and its relationship to culture emergent.
7. Describe ritual.
8. Discuss the interrelationship of ritual with biological factors.
9. Describe the importance of ritual in healing.
10. List and define five universal values.
11. Discuss the importance of values in culture emergent.
12. Describe the change processes that affect culture.
13. Discuss the importance of cultural continuity.
14. Define race and ethnicity.
15. Discuss the limitations of race and ethnicity as concepts for describing culture.

THE STORY OF LIA LEE

We introduce the story of the Lee family here and begin each subsequent chapter with additional information about their encounters with United States medical and social service systems. Their story, as told by Fadiman (1997), highlights many of the important issues of intercultural encounters. In keeping with Sue's (2000) recommended strategies for effective intercultural interaction, we first outline some important background information about Hmong culture and its expression in the early experiences of the Lee family as they found their way to the United States.

- As you read these vignettes in each chapter, consider these questions: How do you think you would react if the Lees were referred to you? How do you think the Lees might react to your typical professional interventions? What might improve the odds of obtaining an outcome that would be best for Lia Lee?

Nao Kao Lee and his wife, Foua Yang, are Hmong refugees now living in the Central Valley of California. The story of their experiences with the medical system in the United States is one that provides profound lessons about the centrality of culture to beliefs, behaviors, and ultimately to outcomes of health care interventions.

To understand fully the story of the Lees, one must begin by reviewing Hmong history and culture. The Hmong are an ancient people who originated in Eurasia and traveled through Siberia to China. The group maintained its separation from other cultures in the countries in which it found itself and experienced considerable persecution because those countries did not understand the Hmong. By 400 AD, the Hmong established themselves in the Honan, Hupeh, and Hunan provinces of China, although they had limited interaction with the Chinese who surrounded them. In their own culture, dislike of authority was pronounced, so the kings who ruled had very limited power. The Hmong were known for not taking orders, not liking to lose, and not being frightened when surrounded by superior numbers.

The Chinese spent many years attempting to overthrow the Hmong power structure and succeeded after 500 years. The Hmong did not accept defeat well, and many conflicts occurred over the years until the beginning of the 19th century, when many Hmong fled China for Vietnam, then Laos and finally, Thailand. They settled in the highlands, an area found inhospitable by other groups. There they continued their tradition of scratching out a living through agriculture while maintaining their separation from the surrounding cultures, a practice that caused continued conflict, especially with the French, who became involved in Indochina in the 19th century.

During the Vietnam War, the United States, by way of the Central Intelligence Agency, enlisted the help of the Hmong because of their history as fierce fighters who had little loyalty to the countries in which they lived. In return for their help, the Hmong were promised assistance. When the United States lost the war, the Hmong were again persecuted, many of them ending up in refugee camps from which large numbers eventually emigrated to the United States.

Among the places in which large numbers of Hmong have settled is Merced, CA. The Lees were part of this group. With them came seven of 13 children; the other six had died. Twelve had been born in Laos, one in a refugee camp in Thailand. The Lees had their 14th child, Lia, in Merced. At age 3 months, Lia had a severe seizure that brought the Lees into contact with the United States medical system, profoundly changing the family and affecting the system as well.

Summarized from Fadiman, A. (1997). *The spirit catches you and you fall down*. New York: Noonday Press.

INTRODUCTION

Culture has many definitions, as you saw in the introduction to this book. For health care providers, finding a concise definition is less important than finding a definition that facilitates effective interaction in clinical situations. This chapter provides a functional definition that can be used to conceptualize culture as it affects and is affected by health care encounters. Moreover, it describes important constructs related to culture that are central to clinical encounters.

OUR MODEL OF CULTURE EMERGENT

We focus on culture as experienced by individuals as it emerges through interaction in complex societies. The term **culture emergent** underscores the processes of change and **adaptation** in learning and using culture.

Our model of culture emergent emphasizes the following:

- Culture is learned. It is transmitted from one generation to the next. Observation and discourse are the primary means of cultural transmission. One learns culture through interaction with others: by listening to, observing, and assessing those interactions. Because culture is learned, it is shared with those from whom it is learned and with those who learn it from you.

- Culture is localized. Culture is formed through discrete interactions with specific individuals. It is from such interactions that one draws meaningful elements that will be shared with some but not all individuals within society (Sherzer, 1987; Urban, 1991). Thus, culture is situated in personally meaningful locales. Interactions in multiple social settings provide multiple contexts for learning culture.

- Culture is patterned. Patterning is essential for social behavior and the development and maintenance of societies. It is essential that individuals develop patterns for behavior that minimize ambiguity and do not require renegotiation of every interaction. Patterns emerge from the repetition of specific samples of behavior and talk. Repeated patterns establish the normal and customary expectations that structure interactions.

- Culture is evaluative. **Values** are embedded in culture and are reflected in individual behavioral decisions and choices. Values reflect the underlying organization of shared structures that facilitate social interaction. Society would not be possible without a significant level of shared values. However, individuals are continuously reconsidering those values in terms of personal relevance. Sometimes, contradictory values may exist, and decisions about which one to acknowledge are contingent on context.

- Culture is persistent but incorporates change. In general, cultural identity is stable, but the cultural knowledge of an individual continues to change over the life course as one encounters new objects, situations, and ideas in one's personal environment. These experiences serve to shape a unique person; however, across society, many individuals may experience the forces for change almost simultaneously and respond in similar ways.

The theoretical framework of culture emergent takes into account the interactions of individuals and their cultural development as well as the process of change in culture over time. Thus, the focus is away from cultural group or cultural mindset and toward individuals making choices within culturally defined boundaries. Culture emergent theory assumes that cultural patterns are dynamic and collectively negotiated through individual interactions, primarily through talk but also by other behavior. It also assumes that much of culture derives from the social, problem-solving, task orientation of human beings.

Our approach to culture allows us to conceptualize culture as a cognitive model of reality as the rules-based approach to culture does. The cognitive model we envision, however, is not static. Instead, it is based upon the cumulative learning experiences of the individual. The model is not a unitary one shared by, and desirable for, everyone in society. It is differentiated and located within individuals. Some elements of culture may be shared with one set of individuals, whereas other elements may be shared with other sets of individuals. Because all individuals have had different experiences in life, personal models always vary at least slightly, even among individuals who live in similar environments and have shared many similar experiences. Moreover, because individuals continue to have new experiences throughout their lives, our model incorporates the notion that culture is ever-changing.

Consider the case of multiple siblings. They may share, in general, similar environmental circumstances during early life, but, typically, siblings are different from each other, often dramatically. Many factors might account for these differences. Genetic inheritance, which provides the foundations for physical appearance, personality, and a host of other significant characteristics, is never identical for non-twin siblings. Birth order is a key environmental characteristic, always unique for each child. Parenting behavior is affected by learning and by circumstance (e.g., economic conditions, new neighborhoods, illness), and subsequent children may receive somewhat different sorts of training. Once children begin to form their own friendships, their experiences, values, and behaviors may diverge quite substantially. Some, but not all, of these factors are cultural.

Care must be taken not to assume that everything is related to culture. The basic test to determine if a factor has a cultural basis is to assess whether the item in question is a learned trait and widely shared among members of a group in contact with each other. In the remainder of this chapter we discuss each of the components of our model of culture emergent and offer examples of their relevance for health care professionals.

Q 2-1. Take a moment to think about culture in relation to your own identification. The theory of culture emergent suggests that your personal experiences in multiple cultures lead to a unique cultural identification for you. Reflect on the cultural identification you selected in Chapter 1. What are some specific examples of ways in which that cultural background affects how you think and behave?

2-2. Think about your experiences with persons from other cultural backgrounds. What other places have you lived or traveled? Have any of these experiences affected your perceptions, values, or behaviors? Are there any obvious cultural influences you have gained from these experiences? (Some common examples of cultural influence are food preferences, articles of clothing, or what you believe about religion, so especially consider those domains.)

CULTURE IS LEARNED

Enculturation is the acquisition of cultural knowledge that allows one to function as a member of a particular society. For example, at an early age,

you learn about appropriate foods, attitudes toward work and leisure, even how to handle pain. You also learn what constitutes appropriate social behaviors and how to distinguish categories of social relationships. You learn to distinguish family members from non-relatives and within the family, aunts, uncles, and cousins from parents and siblings. At present, you are learning the culture of your profession through a process of enculturation embedded in professional education and experience. You learn how to be a health care provider or therapist in part from observing and modeling the behaviors of more experienced providers during clinical experiences and the early years of your career.

Observation and discourse are the primary methods of learning culture. Some enculturation is purposeful (i.e., it is intentionally taught). Elders purposefully teach some elements of culture to children, and schools exist for the purpose of formal cultural transmission. Other elements are not explicitly taught but are acquired from experience, interaction, and the evaluative responses of others. Many elements are learned from peers during informal interaction. For example, when you were in high school, you learned how to dress and act in order to be accepted into your peer group, but no one gave you a specific lecture about how to behave in order to be part of that group. Some cultural lessons (e.g., personal hygiene, attitudes about time) are learned at an early age; others (e.g., appropriate political strategies, how to be a good grandparent) are learned later in life (Figure 2-1).

These learned cultural elements are continuously subject to evaluation. This constant reappraisal is necessary because there may be more than one culturally appropriate behavior available to an individual. During high school, once you learned the rules, you had to make decisions about which style of dress was most comfortable for you and most likely to gain approval from the group from which you sought acceptance. As an adult you must choose among such acceptable alternatives as being a vegetarian or an omnivore by evaluating several available value-laden arguments about health, the environment, the sanctity of life, and the dictates of religion.

Culture is absolutely not genetic. Humans are born with the capacity to think and acquire language and thus, to develop culture, but no one is born with a propensity to a particular cultural array. Every newborn enters the world with a clean cultural slate, a *tabula rasa*. It is possible for parents in New York to adopt a baby from China who will conform perfectly to the cultural expectations of other

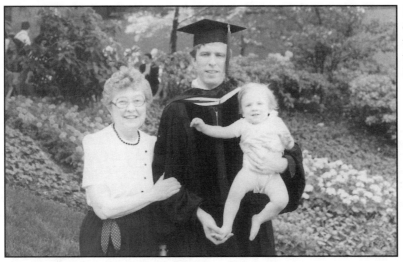

Figure 2-1. This grandmother and father begin early to teach the next generation their cultural value: the importance of education.

New Yorkers as he or she matures. However, if the parents want their child to maintain his or her cultural heritage and deliberately expose the child to language, religion, food, art, and other things Chinese, those experiences will provide the child with knowledge, options, and patterns of behavior that will not be common to most New Yorkers. The child may even develop a **bicultural** sense of self or display multiple sets of cultural identities, depending on context.

Q 2-3. Think of someone you know (or know of)—it could be you—who is bi- or multicultural. What are the cultures involved? What are the sources of the different cultural influences? When are some influences dominant over the others? How much does the person seem to identify with the various cultural influences in his or her background?

Though evolutionary processes facilitate the biological adaptation of small homogeneous communities to extreme environments, this kind of **genetic adaptation** may or may not influence culture. For example, there have been biological adaptations by populations living in arctic cold and at high altitudes. This kind of genetic adaptation may relate to some aspects of culture (e.g., food, clothing, housing, economy) because people must make use of what is available in their environment. However, an Andean potato farmer who is physically well-suited for living at high altitudes can move to Lima, become a professor, and run for president of Peru, or move to the United States, study physics, and become an engineer.

Because culture is learned, it also is shared. You share culture with those from whom you learned it and with those to whom you teach it. In addition, each interaction with another individual provides an opportunity for learning culture and reinforcing elements already acquired. This interactive sharing and mutual reinforcement has the effect of binding you to others and to the group. This process also means that culture is dynamic, with the potential for change.

The transmission process, which is at the heart of sharing, is facilitated by linguistic interaction. What makes two individuals cohere in a society is their shared knowledge of the world. In effect, like attracts like. The discourse produced by one individual is transmitted and copied—the copy being a replica of the original (Urban, 1991). The nature of the transmission process brings us to the second characteristic of our model of culture emergent.

CULTURE IS LOCALIZED

Within a society there may be many groups; an individual may have more or less access to some of these. However, an individual's cultural knowledge emerges through interactions with specific individuals. This is what is meant by **localization**: culture is always situated in personally meaningful, interactive locations. It is from such interactions in your immediate surroundings that you learn meaningful elements that will be shared with some but not all individuals within society. Professional settings offer a kind of well-defined environment for the emergence of localized knowledge. For example, knowing how the nurses' station is set up or how supplies are classified or which music particular surgeons prefer all constitute local knowledge that organizes staff behavior in a hospital and is learned largely through experience or observation. It is not shared with people outside the organization or even with those who work on a different floor or in a different specialty.

Q

2-4. Think about a professional context with which you are familiar. Can you give an example of a site- or profession-specific type of knowledge? How did you acquire that knowledge? How is that knowledge exhibited?

Urban (1991) made a similar point in his discourse-centered approach to culture. According to Urban, the collection of events from which meanings are drawn is publicly accessible. That collection of events is the basis for recognizing interconnections. However, the interconnections are recognized in different ways by individuals, depending in part on the degree and kind of access they have had to the overall community history. Figure 2-2 shows how differently a familiar activity may be enacted in another culture. One consequence is that interactions in multiple social settings provide multiple cultural contexts for the individual.

For our model of culture emergent it is important to note that in complex societies embodying diverse cultural traditions, an individual may draw elements from any number of groups. Note in Figures 2-3 and 2-4 how a familiar object can be used very differently in different cultures.

Moreover, individuals constantly renegotiate their individual identities. Everyone is a bundle of cultural threads, and social context influences individual choices about displaying one or another of them. You may choose, for example, not to disclose your religious affiliation, political party, or sexual orientation to coworkers, whereas some or all of these facets of your identity may be known to family members or close friends outside of work. Sometimes, persons who can choose among several ethnic identities—biracial children, for instance—display one in school settings and another at summer camp. In every interaction, only part of an individual's identity is being exhibited. Therefore, we can never have complete data about another person. To gather information, we must ask questions, observe, develop strategies of interaction, initiate behaviors, and move on. This situation is especially pronounced in constrained settings, such as health care interactions, where time available for interaction and appropriate behaviors is extremely circumscribed.

Q

2-5. Think about the ways in which you display the varied facets of your cultural identity. Make a short list of settings in which you might emphasize one aspect over another (e.g., holiday celebrations, work settings, child-related events, and so on). For each one, identify the part of your cultural identification that is most salient. Think about why you choose to behave the way you do.

The localized nature of culture is what makes it personally meaningful. The meaning assigned to any cultural component reflects the perspective of the individual. At any moment in time each individual is responding to a particular view of an interaction. We call this view or perspective **vantage**, a concept discussed more fully in Chapter 5. Here, it is sufficient to appreciate that meaning is created from the perspective of an individual's own vantage and that vantage itself is a complex association of elements, some cultural and some not.

To understand the localization of culture, it is helpful to understand the nature of social organization. Status positions and social roles are the building blocks of social organization. We use a discussion of these societal components to illustrate how culture is localized.

Culture and Society

In popular usage, the terms **culture** and **society** are often used interchangeably. The two are related, as in many cases the people of a given society share much of the same culture. Thus, the precise meanings of the terms are not always apparent. It may help if you think about society as the organization of people, whereas culture is the more or less shared understandings that provide meaning to peoples' lives.

A society is an association of individuals who form a cohesive unit, at least along some significant dimensions. All societies are organized in the sense that the interactions of the individuals are highly patterned. Human societies are structured around institutions. Institutions are patterns of behavior organized around a central theme.

There are some types of institutions that are found universally in human societies: economic and political systems, the family, and religion. Such institutions are **universal** because all people have

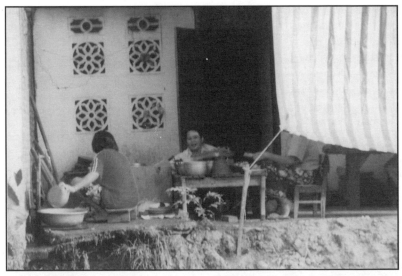

Figure 2-2. Cooking takes place outdoors in rural Thailand. Photo courtesy of Wendy Schmidt.

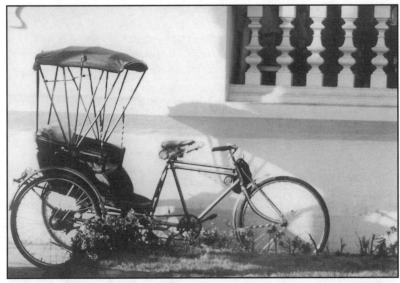

Figure 2-3. A bicycle is being used as a rickshaw in Thailand. Photo courtesy of Wendy Schmidt.

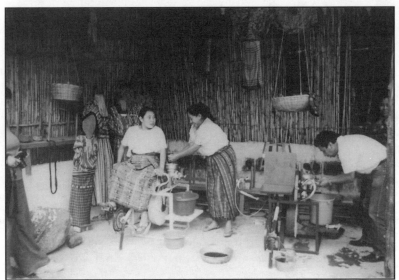

Figure 2-4. Here a bicycle is used as a corn-mill in Guatemala.

many of the same basic individual and social needs. People everywhere need to solve problems related to getting food and shelter, raising children, ensuring security and stability, transmitting knowledge, coping with change, and explaining unfair or unfortunate happenstance. Other kinds of institutions, such as those organized for formal education, the military, and sports, are found in many but not all societies.

There are a few **cultural universals**—rules, concepts, and strategies for meeting needs that are found in every human group. For example, people everywhere sort individuals by age and sex, and they tend to differentiate status positions and social roles. However, the specifics of such distinctions vary widely from one society to another.

Q 2-6. Think about the ways in which people are sorted in your community. Which of the following factors seem to be involved: wealth, place of residence, level of education, membership in a particular clan or family, profession, number of children, marital status, dress, type of car owned? What other sorting factors can you identify?

Status Positions

Status refers to a position in society with certain rights and obligations. You simultaneously occupy several different status positions, each with particular rights and obligations. Status positions can be categorized as either **ascribed** or **achieved**.

Ascribed status is one that you acquire by being born into it. Ascribed status positions include those that result from your age, sex, or kinship. For example, daughter/son, sister/brother, and cousin are ascribed status positions. Moreover, if you were born into a royal family, you also might have the ascribed status of prince or princess.

Achieved status is one that you acquire through special effort or competition. Physical therapist, Sunday school teacher, and Kiwanis Club member are examples of achieved status positions; so are student, football player, social worker, and part-time sales clerk.

It is important to acknowledge that some statuses that people consider to be products of their achievements, such as educational attainment, professional rewards, or financial success, actually result in part from the luck of one's birth. Gender, race, and social class all restrict some elements of potential achievement. Family connections, disability status, personality, opportunity, and physical appearance may all be factors in narrowing or broadening access to achievement. And, in cases of cultural difference, achieved statuses may not translate well across the cultural boundary. Countless refugee or immigrant physicians, attorneys, pharmacists, physicists, or engineers have ended up as laboratory technicians, janitors, day-care and landscape workers, or in other low-prestige occupations, with their achievements obscured or denied. It is well for health care providers to be aware, first of their own status rankings and, then, of the possibility of misinterpretation of status across cultural groups.

If you took the total list of status positions for a society and organized the positions by identifying whose rights affected the obligations of others, by social power and prestige or by access to economic resources, you would have a good idea of social relations in that society. Such an arrangement of status positions would produce a representation of the society's **social structure**. In our society it would be an impossible task to list every status position and relate each one to all the others, but we can approximate the social structure by selecting representative status positions that reflect a specialized part of society.

Q 2-7. Think about the status positions you occupy. List some in the margin. Now decide whether each one is ascribed or achieved.

By examining status positions and their rights and obligations, the relative position of elected and appointed officials in government can be charted, and large businesses frequently diagram the lines of authority within their organization. These diagrams are usually called a table of organization or organizational chart. In reality, they represent pieces of society's social structure. Obviously, the task of diagramming all the status positions constituting the social structure in a small agricultural group would be easier than trying to diagram that of a large, **complex society** such as that of the entire United States.

As an example, consider the diagram of positions in a hospital (see box on page 25). Each person has a clear relationship to others in the organization. Some have supervisor/supervisee relationships; others are expected to interact but do not have reporting relationships to each other. Generally, level of responsibility, economic rewards, and prestige all increase with positions that are higher in the hospital hierarchy. Conversely, posi-

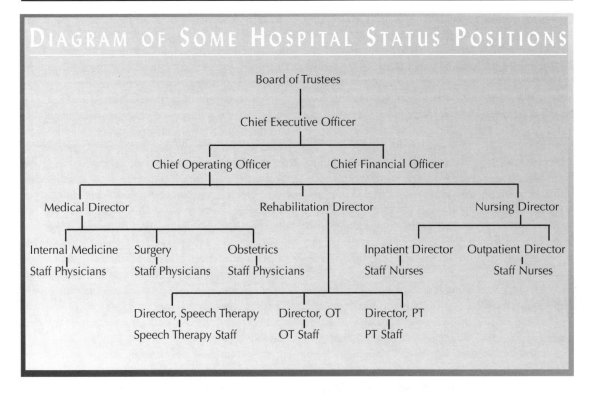

DIAGRAM OF SOME HOSPITAL STATUS POSITIONS

tions on the same horizontal level are approximately equivalent for these variables. However, there may be considerable variation among individuals within a single position. For example, tenure and skill level, as well as personal characteristics, may result in variations of economic rewards or prestige among staff therapists.

Q 2-8. Examine the hospital organization chart in the box above. How well does this chart conform to your own experience of hospital organization? What are some of the behavioral or interactional markers of the different statuses? How does a new employee learn about these different statuses? How does a patient learn to identify persons of different status?

Identifying and distinguishing status positions is one of the primary functions of socialization; normal social relations could not be maintained if members of a society did not agree on what constitutes a status position and what are the rights and obligations of that position. Status positions are not the same in all societies, although they exist in all societies, and thus can be defined and described for all societies. For example, the status positions within a kinship system may vary from one culture to the next. Perhaps a grandparent is owed more respect in one culture than another. Moreover, a status posi-

tion that exists in one kinship system (e.g., parallel cousin) has no meaning in a culture that does not distinguish between mothers' brothers' children and mothers' sisters' children.

Status positions evolve over time as specialization and the ways of differentiating people increase. Hunter-gatherer societies have relatively few status positions, whereas agricultural and industrial societies have greater numbers of status positions. In highly complex societies, entire systems of status positions can exist, determining the behavior of enormous numbers of people, and yet can be unknown by members of the society who are outside the particular system. Some examples include the hierarchy of Roman Catholic clergy, military officers, or hospital personnel.

Many status positions are reciprocal; that is, they come in pairs. For example, you cannot be a niece without having an aunt or uncle, nor can you be an aunt without a niece or nephew. The same is true for employer and employee, clinician and client, and many other status positions.

2-9. Think for a moment about the rights and responsibilities you have, or will have, as a health care professional. Jot a few notes in the margin to help you recall your ideas as you read further. What responsibilities do you assign your clients? What are their rights? What can they expect of you? **Q**

Reciprocal status positions such as health care recipient and provider involve reciprocal rights and obligations. As a health care recipient, you have the right to expect the provider to listen to your concerns and to be competent to treat you or to refer you to the appropriate provider. You have the right to expect the provider to respect your dignity and privacy and to maintain confidentiality about what you report. You have the right to expect the provider to see you at the appointed time and to be responsive to emergencies, especially if they are life-threatening. At the same time, you have the responsibility to report your concerns accurately and comprehensively, to be prompt for appointments, to adhere to the agreed upon treatment, to report results, and to pay for care in a timely fashion.

As a health care provider, you have the right to expect care recipients to show up for appointments, to provide you with accurate information about their conditions and concerns, and to provide payment. You have the responsibility to acquire current knowledge and skills, to be aware of and communicate your limitations, to make appropriate referrals, to respect the confidentiality of information provided by the recipient, to adhere as closely as possible to a designated schedule or to inform the recipient of reasons for delays, and to provide the appropriate treatment, neither more nor less.

Notice how the rights of one reciprocal status position tend to define the obligations of the other. The same is true for niece and aunt or any other pair of reciprocal status positions. This balancing of rights and obligations helps clarify expectations so that you know what to expect of other people, as well as how you should behave with them.

Q 2-10. Think further about your professional identity. How well did your list of rights and responsibilities correspond to those we outline here? Use the margin to list some of your current professional status positions. How will these change when you graduate from your professional education or are promoted to the higher position in your status hierarchy? What adjustments do you think you will have to make to accommodate the anticipated changes?

Social Roles

A **social role** is the behavior expected as appropriate for a specific status position in a particular situation. Thus, for the status positions of student and professor, knowing the rights and obligations of the positions, you also know the behaviors that might be expected from individuals in those status positions. You know how a student or a professor ought to behave in normal circumstances.

Of course, not everyone behaves exactly as you might expect, and no one behaves as you expect all the time. Individual personality factors and differences in socialization mean that not everyone has the same understanding of a particular role. Certainly, cultural differences can affect one's understanding of status positions. For example, you might feel comfortable calling a professor by her first name if she invites you to do so, whereas a classmate might find that she is uneasy about doing so because of her own perceptions of faculty–student roles. Graduate students who did undergraduate study outside the United States may have very different ideas about proper student–professor interaction than those who have only attended American schools.

It is remarkable, however, that so many of us behave as we are expected to so much of the time. This consistency is a testament to the power of socialization and the basic genetically grounded sociality of *Homo sapiens* (Carrithers, 1992).

We all occupy a number of different status positions simultaneously: student, spouse, sibling, for example. Correspondingly, we have a number of different roles that we might enact. Usually we maintain these roles in harmony. In fact, in your interactions with others, you expect them to have multiple obligations, just as you do. Thus you appreciate a friend's need to tend to a sick child instead of keeping a date with you or an employee's decision to attend a funeral rather than make a sales call.

It is essential to recognize that statuses and role definitions change, with the result that institutionalized patterns of behavior within a society change. For example, the status position of father in our society began to change significantly for many individuals in the decades after World War II. The rights (e.g., household authority) and obligations (e.g., sole monetary provider) changed and thus the role (i.e., how fathers are expected to behave) changed. The ultimate result was a change in the institution of the family because the statuses and roles of all family members changed in response to each other. No one directed this change. It was not dictated by the government or by psychologists or social workers. This change came about because many individuals reached a new understanding of their options in life and what needed to be done to take advantage of the opportunities at hand.

Role Conflict

The fact that everyone holds multiple status positions simultaneously can lead to confusion. Moreover, even when we do not experience a change in status, our perceptions and expectations of others may change over time as we get to know them better, in a different way, under different circumstances, or when we learn about additional status positions they may have.

Suppose, for example, that you move into a new neighborhood and the woman next door seems bright, helpful, and friendly, and you have a pleasant conversation about the weather, plants growing in the yard, and other somewhat superficial subjects suitable to interaction with a new acquaintance. You enjoy your neighbor and look forward to getting to know her better gradually, over the course of time. A few days later, you go to the physical therapy clinic to which you have been referred. The therapist asks a series of personal questions about the nature of your injury and its impact on your work, home, and sexual functioning—issues you are usually somewhat reticent to discuss. The physical therapist is your next door neighbor.

Although the roles of therapist and neighbor are not incompatible (after all, therapists have to be neighbors to someone), the relationship between you two may change. The status positions you and the therapist occupy do not change, but the enhanced understanding of the complex roles she has may alter your behavior toward her, as well as her behavior toward you. Both you and the therapist are likely to experience discomfort in the situation. This discomfort results from **role conflict**.

We all experience role conflict. We all occupy multiple roles with differing demands, and sometimes the demands of one role are in conflict with those of another. Role conflict results from the fact that others hold conflicting expectations of you, and no matter how you behave in a given situation, you cannot meet everyone's expectations.

During much of our lives, we are placed in situations of role conflict, and the result inevitably is personal discomfort. Consider the dilemma of a social worker in child protective services who is also a wife and mother of small children. Imagine her receiving an emergency call to deal with a situation of an abused child in her work role on a Saturday that happens to be her young daughter's birthday. Does she go in to her office immediately to deal with the abused child, or does she stay at home and spend this important day with her own child? Does she seek some kind of compromise, arranging to go to the office immediately after her daughter's party?

To be a good friend and not disappoint another friend by going to the movie with him tonight, or to be a good student and study for tomorrow's test? To be a good employee, always working overtime, or to be a good husband and father? Citizen, church member, scout leader, neighbor, youth volunteer—all of these statuses may compete for your time and energy, and inevitably, there will be conflicts. How you resolve these conflicts may be a measure of your social maturity and your ability to balance the demands of life in your world. The choices you make may result from deep-seated values related to your enculturation.

As a health care provider, you want to establish rapport with your clients or patients and take the time necessary for a full evaluation. Conversely, you also need to generate income for the institution that employs you. There is an inherent dilemma in every clinical encounter that can be viewed as role conflict between being a treatment provider and being a revenue producer. Ultimately, the resolution hinges on appropriate time allocation, but reaching that resolution may require accommodation between the two roles and the values they imply.

2-11. Students sometimes experience role conflict **Q** when they begin their clinical or internship experiences. They are surprised to find that they are now "authority figures" to the patients they serve while still being students to their professors. Have you experienced similar role conflicts? Can you recall specific examples? How did you deal, or how might you deal, with this challenging situation?

The Individual in Society

Even though we are all influenced by society, by our interactions with other individuals, and by the structures that have arisen in our particular society, it is clear that we each remain individual agents. It is as individuals that we assign meaning to particular behaviors, even if those behaviors are social behaviors common within a group. Moreover, as individuals, we each have our own biology, in part genetically encoded at conception, and in part the result of biological history. This issue is discussed more fully in Chapter 3.

How society regulates individual conduct is a classic problem in the social sciences. Urban (1991) suggests that **regulation** is accomplished

by slipping normative messages about how individuals ought to behave into speech in

Figure 2-5. Many cultures have specific rituals related to marriage. Photo courtesy Robert Good Photography.

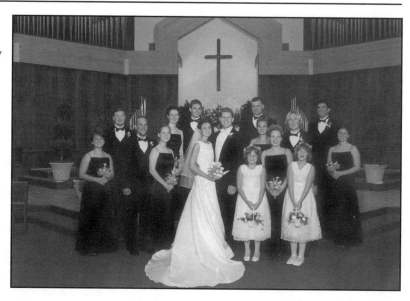

such a way that the message can be inferred. The message is suspended in the realm between consciousness and unawareness and appears not as a rule imposed from the outside, but rather as part of the social being of the individual, as self-regulation. (p. 67)

For example, parents routinely choose which of their children's behaviors to acknowledge with a hug, which with a frown.

Q 2-12. Consider your own behavior. How do you regulate, by words or gestures, the behavior of others? For example, how do you indicate to a friend that a personal question is too intrusive? To an acquaintance that a joke is offensive? To an instructor that you do not understand an assignment? Can you think of similar examples of how others—a spouse, child, coworker, boss, or friend—regulate your behavior?

At this point, we are not concerned about the specific mechanism by which normative behavior is established. For our model of culture emergent, it is sufficient to posit that it occurs through social interactions. Moreover, because the efficiency of interactions is a prerequisite for the development of a society, it is essential that individuals develop patterns for behavior that minimize ambiguity about relationships and roles. Patterned behaviors, with recognizable and recurring components, promote comfort, efficiency, and continuity in cultural practice. In other words, as individuals we develop patterns of social familiarity, grounded in reciprocity and an individual history of experience.

CULTURE IS PATTERNED

Culture is patterned in two senses. First, it is patterned in that the components of culture are integrated, reflecting a generalizable pattern for individual action. Secondly, culture is patterned in the repetitive behaviors of individuals, which become so ingrained they seem like empirical reality. One form these patterns take is the rituals that characterize a culture.

What Is Ritual?

We may think of **ritual** as patterned, repeated, formalized behaviors enacted by individuals but sanctioned by groups. Historically, ritual has been equated with ceremony—the occurrence or use of ritual in social situations involving two or more individuals. Some commonly observed rituals include weddings (Figure 2-5), funerals, and special holiday meals, but each culture has specialized rituals, such as the high school prom, the Super Bowl, or standardized examinations. The term also has been used to indicate idiosyncratic behaviors, as when we speak of the personal rituals performed by swimmers before a meet, baseball players before a game or when going to bat, or surgeons during an operation. Some theorists have insisted that ritual always has a sacred quality (Gluckman & Gluckman, 1977), but the difficulty of defining "sacred" makes this analysis somewhat ambiguous.

Chapple and Coon (1942) defined ritual as a symbolic configuration used to restore equilibrium after a crisis (p. 398):

When a person is born, comes to puberty, gets married, becomes ill, suffers bodily injury, dies or is initiated into a new institution, his relations to other members of his group are necessarily changed. The process of change in the interaction rates, upsetting the equilibria of the individuals concerned, is countered by a series of techniques requiring the interactions of the disturbed individuals in specific and habitual ways. If the rituals are associated with the crises derived from the actions of a single individual, they are called **rites of passage**.

Life cycle events, such as weddings, bar mitzvahs, and birthdays, are rites of passage and center on the individual. These events commemorate personal changes in status or social identity. Although many members of the group may engage in the same ritual expressions, particular occasions are associated with the individual person or cohort experiencing them. They publicly alter, or confirm the alteration of, an individual's relationship to the rest of the society.

Q 2-13. What was the most recent life cycle ritual in which you participated? Were you the focal individual for whom the ritual was performed, or were you an observer and member of the group to which the individual belonged? What were the major parts of the ritual, and what were they meant to communicate to the focal individual about his or her changed status in the community?

Another type of ritual involves the whole group. These rituals, sometimes called **calendrical rituals** and termed **rites of intensification** by Chapple and Coon, often result from or commemorate changes in the environment. They serve to confirm, strengthen, and display group membership and identity. Thanksgiving, family reunions, midnight mass on Christmas Eve, the Veterans' Day parade, block parties, and the World Series are all types of rites of intensification. They commemorate and confirm group membership (as Americans, or family, or Catholics, or veterans, or neighbors, or fans) and contribute to cultural cohesion.

Q 2-14. Think about a ritual activity that you engage in with other people on a regular schedule. Where, when, and with whom do you participate? What is the origin of the ritual? What effect does it have on members of the group? What makes it a rite of intensification?

Chapple and Coon (1942) viewed all ritual, even ritual affecting an entire group, as having a locus within the individual, for it is the individual who is affected by the crisis. Recall the Lee family (Fadiman, 1997) introduced at the beginning of this chapter. The Lees experienced multiple changes in environment, from the mountains of Laos to a refugee camp to an apartment in Merced, California. One of their reactions to the changes was to employ rituals familiar to their culture to re-establish equilibrium in each setting. For example, they used particular rituals to welcome each new child into the family. These ritual forms were not familiar to the non-Hmong residents of Merced, but they were the customary observances, developed over centuries of history, that enabled the Hmong people in general, and the Lees in particular, to maintain a sense of cultural continuity even in the midst of changed circumstances. They were important elements of family cohesion and cultural identity.

Ritual and the Coordination of Social and Biological Systems

Chapple's (1970) perspective has continued to evolve. In 1970 he theorized that ritual events may entrain biological rhythms. It may be that biological rhythms are synchronized through ritual to respond to environmental exigencies and stresses. These rituals may reduce variability of behavior and increase the probability that predetermined, or practical, patterns will occur. Ritual behavior may enable individuals to attend selectively to critical stimuli (e.g., making a free throw in basketball) and to ignore or de-emphasize other stimuli (e.g., crowd noise) that might interfere with performance (Miracle & Southard, 1993). Lex (1979) assumed a similar position, stating that "the *raison d'être* for rituals is the readjustment of dysphasic biological and social rhythms by manipulation of neurophysiological structures under controlled conditions" (p. 144). Thus, the entire body may receive repetitive, patterned information that affects biological rhythms in conjunction with the autonomic nervous system. Likewise, biological events such as illness may alter rituals, or at least their enactment by specific individuals.

Wallace (1966) was among the first to attend theoretically to the importance of individual behaviors as rituals. Wallace identified two distinct but parallel functions of ritual: social ritual that coordinates the interactions of individuals and personal ritual that coordinates an individual's own biological systems. Laughlin, McManus, and d'Aquili (1992) state that ritual behavior is patterned, repet-

THE SUCKING CURE

A **shaman** is a type of specialized healer commonly found in many traditional cultures in North and South America. Shamans mix practical remedies and advice with abstractions, often couched in stories, songs, and dance. They may also heal by diverting attention from the problem. Much of a shaman's success derives from the manipulation of "a coherent system of symbolic communication" shared with his or her patients (Sharon, 1978). The shaman uses symbols to help patients connect their individual situations with the universal. In contemporary parlance, it might be said that shamans empower their patients through the power of positive thinking. As a culture evolves or encounters forces for change, a shaman may combine the traditional and modern elements into a new system that is fully functional in the contemporary world (Sharon, 1978).

One of the most widespread curing practices used by Andean shamans in South America is the "sucking cure." The sucking cure is based on the belief that an individual becomes sick when the balance of the natural is upset. When foreign spirit or matter enters a person's body, it violates the harmony of the body and adverse symptoms appear. If the foreign entity can be removed, natural balance will be restored and the individual will become well. In such situations, the shaman may attempt to remove the foreign entity by sucking it out of the patient's body.

When a sucking cure is to be performed, the patient's family is assembled. The family is necessarily present because it is believed that the individual is an extension of the family and family members may be part of the affliction as well as the cure. Moreover, the addition of family members' energies and concentration increases the power available for the shaman to focus on the healing process. Family members may serve as drummers or perform other essential roles in the curing ritual. In this way, all of those most affected by the sickness (i.e., the patient and the patient's family) work to facilitate their own healing.

After a careful diagnosis of the patient and the use of practical efforts such as massage, herbs, and other remedies, the shaman will prepare for the sucking cure. To perform this cure, the shaman must enter a deep trance. This state may be achieved through dance and the use of percussion music, which is produced by drums, rattles, and bells, or through the use of drugs such as tobacco or hallucinogens.

The passage into this altered state is the **shamanic path**—that way of seeing and knowing which is hidden to ordinary members of the community. It is in this altered state that the shaman, who becomes the vessel for the supernatural, will effect the cure of the sick patient. By sucking out the invasive foreign entity, the shaman can restore nature's balance. When this task has been accomplished, the shaman may spit out the offending entity, or at least its material manifestation, in order to demonstrate to the patient and the attending family that the cure is complete.

Adapted from Miracle, A. W. (1997). A shaman to organizations. In C. R. Ember, M. Ember, & P. N. Peregrine (Eds.), *Research frontiers in anthropology* (Vol. 1, pp. 133-150). Englewood Cliffs, NJ: Prentice Hall.

itive, and structured to produce inter- or intra-organismic coordination. These insights are important for health providers because any activity involving biological and social systems has the potential to affect health behaviors and outcomes. Health care itself has many rituals, from admission or intake procedures to introduction of staff to patient to treatment planning.

Q 2-15. What are some rituals of your profession? How might these rituals appear to someone unfamiliar with them?

We are only beginning to understand the biological bases of ritual. In the past, most social scientists have focused on the social functions of ritual, but ritual clearly has a biological base within individuals. Humans are born with a capacity for ritual, and as individuals we invent it and use it for specific effects, such as hitting a baseball, doing well on a test, or remembering to take daily medications. We also are subject to the effects of ritual devised by others in efforts to control our behaviors and emotional states. Ritual occurs at the nexus of biological, social, and psychological forces and incorporates both individual and interactive elements. Ritual is an important locus for observing culture, as it is such an important expression of culturally embedded behaviors. It is crucial for health care providers to be aware of ritual and its importance. Health and illness are targets for ritual behavior in every cultural group, and ritual can play an important role in the way clients perceive and comply with treatment options.

Ritual and Healing

What does ritual mean to health care providers? As highly patterned, repetitive behaviors, rituals are a significant mechanism for the transmittal of culture. Rituals are not only cultural lessons to be learned, but their performance is a means of replication. One masters the sensorimotor aspects of ritual in an effort to control one's own behavior in a way that has been learned in a traditional context. Ritual helps perpetuate the meaningful past and influence the future.

Social ritual is the purest expression of cultural control. It is not subordinated to any other immediate goal than the performance itself. Where the conscious ideology formulates a practical goal for the activity (e.g., the promotion of health or fertility or the bringing of rain), ritual as a means to those ends is nevertheless guided only by the norm of its proper and faithful execution. It is not guided by an immediate practical purpose that might influence the sensorimotor habits themselves. Those habits are regulated only by the past, by tradition, by culture. The success or failure of the ritual is attributed to the perfection with which it has taken place (Urban, 1991, p. 112).

Rituals associated with healing demonstrate both the performance aspect of ritual and how powerful cultural messages within ritual can affect individuals. For example, consider the shamanic ritual that anthropologists call the "sucking cure," described on page 30.

All of the individuals participating in the sucking cure—shaman, patient, and patient's family—must sense that their interests are interdependent and their destinies related before healing is possible. The healer creates a shared vision of health while helping individuals to understand the nature of the illness. However, the cure is effected by the afflicted patient. It is as if the healer is a midwife to a healthier organism.

This notion—that help and healing come from within—is important. In his book *Anatomy of an* *Illness as Perceived by the Patient*, Norman Cousins (1979) quotes Dr. Albert Schweitzer's similar observation: "The witch doctor (i.e., shaman) succeeds for the same reason all the rest of us succeed. Each patient carries his own doctor inside him" (p. 69). It is as if patients hold the answers to their own questions, the solutions to their problems. The shaman is engaged only to help them obtain the vision to see these things within themselves.

Q

2-16. In what ways might physicians be like shamans? In what ways might the healing practices of modern Western medicine be considered healing rituals? To what extent is any health care provider—credentialed, licensed, practicing in a "sacred" space not accessible to outsiders except in a patient role—a kind of ritual specialist?

2-17. Recall Miner's essay about the Nacirema in Chapter 1. Does his description of the "medicine man" make more sense from this perspective?

2-18. What are some rituals in which you engage when sick? What rituals do you observe before or during stressful situations, such as job interviews or examinations?

2-19. Patterned behaviors, including rituals, help shape an evaluative system for assessing one's own and others' behaviors. This evaluative nature of culture is another trait emphasized in our model of culture emergent.

CULTURE IS EVALUATIVE

Values are the systems of categorization that assign moral or ethical judgment to ideas and behaviors. Values are deeply embedded in culture, where they constitute an evaluative system for individual behavioral decisions and choices. Values reflect the underlying organization of shared structures that facilitate social interaction, so many members of a society are likely to have similar values. Moreover, society would not be possible without a significant level of shared values. However, individuals continuously reconsider those values for their degree of personal relevance, creating variations in the patterns of values exhibited by members of society.

One way to establish your social identity is by defining who you are not, a process accomplished through comparative evaluation of the group to which you belong (or one to which you would like to belong) with others. For example, a nurse is not a physician, therapist, or teacher, although his or her role may involve some aspects of the activities performed by these other professionals. The expression of pejorative comparisons can be especially effective, for you simultaneously establish that you are not a member of some other group while relatively elevating the prestige of your own group.

Consider the following example. You probably have heard someone make a comment similar to this one: "Those people don't have jobs because they are lazy." Such an evaluative statement results from viewing others from a distance. Someone making such a statement may not have considered a number of factors. Perhaps the work being performed by "those people" is not recognized by the speaker or is not acknowledged by paid employment. Perhaps there are no culturally suitable jobs available nearby and no transportation available to get to job sites. Perhaps the referent individuals may not have the educational background or skills needed to fill positions that are available. Certainly someone making such a statement has little appreciation of the possible effects of systematic discrimination.

The principal effect of such a statement is to confirm a boundary between the speaker and some other group of people by establishing values—employment, industriousness—that the speaker can claim for him- or herself and deny to those on the other side of the boundary. Such distancing generalizations, although common, are not helpful to the goal of providing culturally effective care. Value judgments are inevitable but can be made explicit and can be evaluated for their utility in a particular circumstance, such as in the treatment room. If the issue is a joint injury, does it really matter whether the patient had a job or not when the injury occurred?

Q 2-20. Think for a moment about the values you rank highly. What is it you value that makes you want to belong to the professional group you are training for or are already a member of? What are the attributes or activities that your chosen profession itself seems to value most highly? How do you think your profession is valued by others? Note your answers in the margin.

Values as an Integrated System

Although there may not be a single definition of values that everyone agrees on, one way to understand values is to observe that they are our concepts of what is desirable and thus serve as criteria for understanding and evaluating behavior. Some values are embedded in religion or another standard of morality. Other values may have nothing to do with religious traditions or teachings, but rather with reproduction of perceived economic or social needs. However, most values are grounded in and reinforced by one or more social institutions, such as economic, political, or family structures. **Value orientation** may be developed through professional education and socialization. For example, professional codes of ethics, such as the Hippocratic oath, convey specific values to which individuals in a profession are expected to conform.

Most people respond to their environment by developing a value orientation that they perceive as being rational and sensible and that will maximize their potential to thrive and perpetuate themselves. A value orientation is reinforced when other people associate an individual with a particular personal orientation and come to expect that individual to behave in a manner consistent with that orientation. In other words, if other people tend to see you as being a "good" person, they will interpret your behavior as being ethical, which in turn reinforces your tendency to act in these expected ways.

However, we often face contradictory moral claims, such as expecting both justice and forgiveness. Given certain social constraints, individuals may choose whether to demand "an eye for an eye" or "to turn the other cheek." This contradiction explains why a person can state a value, illustrate its application in making judgments, identify its boundaries, and then choose to ignore it behaviorally (Williams, 1979). For example, a parent may tell a child that honesty is always the best policy, yet that same parent is unlikely to say to the boss, "Honestly, sir, I believe you are stupid." Thus, when describing the relationship between values and behavior it is preferable to talk about a person's value orientation rather than a discrete set of values. Individuals may not always be perfectly consistent in acting on their values, but they adhere closely enough to a general orientation that their behavior is usually predictable. Of course, a basic level of predictability is essential for stable social relations within society.

Value orientations are determined by one's life experiences. Moreover, it appears that most value orientations are acquired early in life and that most values are acquired before adolescence. Subsequent life events, especially personal crises, may—but rarely do—significantly change our values after adolescence. We may refine our value system as we go along, but our basic value orientation remains much the same.

Socialization within our families and our community is one means of acquiring values. However, socialization is not the same for all members of any society. Gender, age, innate skills, and social position are just some of the variables affecting an individual's socialization experiences. These, in turn, affect the acquisition of values.

For most individuals, the primary socializing influence derives from the previous generation. Parents, teachers, and other potential role models have learned what they believe to be important, practical, necessary, and desirable, and they pass these beliefs along to children—intentionally and otherwise. This process occurs generation after generation, so the cumulative effect influences a society's culture. Because in any society at any given point in time many life experiences may be shared among members, it is to be expected that individuals born about the same time will tend to share some values. That is, those born about the same time constitute age cohorts that are likely to be socialized in similar circumstances, exposed to similar cultural norms, and undergo some similar life experiences. As a result, these individuals may share some common understandings of what constitutes the desirable. It is this fact that allows pundits to identify groups such as "Baby Boomers" or "Generation Xers" as sharing specifically identifiable value orientations.

It should not be supposed that all members of a society are alike. Indeed, no two individuals, even twins, have identical life experiences. We each have different opportunities to experience life and to learn from those experiences. Between identical twins, those differences may not appear great; however, between males and females, rich and poor, urban and rural individuals, and ethnic majorities and minorities, those differences in life experiences could potentially be quite significant. The interaction of individual and cultural factors is considered in greater detail in Chapter 3.

Ideally, there is considerable consensus about values within a society or group, as this common perception is one of the factors that helps glue individuals together in social institutions. However it is doubtful that there ever is total agreement on values, even in small groups. Different cultures, differ-

ent groups within a society, or different individuals within a group may agree or disagree on what is valuable. For example, among physicians, there are individuals who believe strongly in the preservation of life at all costs and others who believe in "death with dignity" and focus more explicitly on **quality of life** over extension of life.

Our values—our concepts of what is desirable—change as we grow older. Your life stage as a child, youth, young adult, middle-aged, or elderly individual may also affect your value orientation. Middle-aged parents may emphasize the values they have acquired over the years when they say to their children, "When you are my age you will understand" or "When I was your age..." At the same time, the child's values may reflect his or her desire to conform to peer group expectations, as children may perceive that such conformity will maximize their potential to thrive in their social situation.

Values are multidimensional. They do not always consist of yes/no or either/or entities. Rather, an individual's value orientation consists of a series of rank-ordered, prioritized options. Usually, most of the options for any specific value category have at least some cultural legitimacy. You might firmly believe that it is best to "forgive and forget." However there might be some violations under specific circumstances that would evoke from you the demand for an eye or a tooth. For example, a person firmly opposed to capital punishment, valuing forgiveness over revenge, may change that opinion when a loved one is murdered. Another person who favors the death penalty may change his or her opinion to value life over punishment after viewing an execution.

The notion that the goal of moral principles is happiness is well-rooted in Western religion and science. Many social scientists believe that morality is central to a scientific theory of human nature. Even Sigmund Freud (1965) maintained that moral principles were so significant that they occupied a fundamental position in his structural model of the mind. Individuals who diverge significantly from prevailing value systems may be stigmatized by others in their social or cultural group.

Our value system connects us to the external world, to other people, and to other communities or cultures. For many individuals, adapting to a changing environment means that value systems lose some of their congruence. In less volatile times, there might be less variation in values and greater congruence with other aspects of life, for the environment would not demand as much flexibility in our behavioral repertoire. Today, most of us can

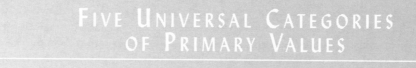

FIVE UNIVERSAL CATEGORIES OF PRIMARY VALUES

1. A conception of the character of innate **human nature**
2. Our **relationship to nature** and the use of technology
3. A temporal focus of human life or **time**
4. A conception of **human activity**
5. A conception of **human relationships** to others

Adapted from Kluckhohn, F. R., & Strodtbeck, F. L. (1961). *Variations in value orientations*. Evanston, IL: Row, Peterson.

only imagine life in a stable environment with little perceptible social change. Now, new technologies rapidly change perceptions, as in the case of new imaging techniques or genetic interventions in health care.

The reason conventional values are not working today... is because the starting assumptions are wrong for modern times. Human values are not absolute; they are not immutably prefixed by natural law or divine ordination. Human values by nature are evolutionary, interrelated, and conditional on the context in which they evolve. To cling to unchanging values in a rapidly changing world can be fatal. (Sperry, 1993, p. 883)

Q 2-21. Can you identify values that you do not share with your parents or your parents' generation? Can you think of ways in which technology has challenged conventional values? (Consider reproductive technologies or freedom of speech values.)

2-22. Can you think of a recent situation in which some of your own values came into conflict, either with each other, with the values of your peers, or with a novel situation that called for a value judgment?

Your behavior, like that of most individuals, is likely to be consistent with your general value orientation. All of your values are interrelated, which allows you to avoid internal value conflicts most of the time. The parts of your value system must work together in order for you to maintain a personal sense of balance, as well as rationality and emotional well-being. Individuals may have very different value systems from one another, but almost everyone has a system of well-integrated, congruent values.

Some Primary Values

Culture is one factor in determining our value systems, and most social scientists recognize that there are differences within and among cultures. Kluckhohn and Strodtbeck (1961) have suggested that there are a limited number of universal categories of primary values that the human species shares.

Culture determines the specific content of each of these categories as well as the range of acceptable variation within each. Culture also helps structure priorities or relative emphases. Of course, individual personality affects prioritization or emphasis. What follows is a brief explanation of each of these five universal categories of primary values.

2-23. Before continuing, take a moment to reflect on your own ideas about each category given in the box above. How would you describe your conception of human nature, nature, time, activity, and relationships with others? Make notes so you can refer to them later. **Q**

Human Nature

There are three logical conceptualizations of the character of innate human nature: evil, neutral or mixed, and good. Related is the question of whether human nature is mutable or immutable; that is, whether it can change. As Kluckhohn and Strodtbeck (1961) have noted, the dominant North American orientation since the time of the Puritans—the view held by Old American culture—has been that human nature is basically evil but perfectible. According to this view, constant control and self-discipline are required if real goodness is to be achieved. However, during the 20th century a growing number of Americans began to accept the idea that human nature is a mixture of good and evil.

Q 2-24. What is your own basic conception of human nature? Do you believe people are basically good?

2-25. In your view, how important are self-control and discipline for a person? Can you recall the sources of your current views on these matters?

Relationship to Nature

What is nature and our relationship to it? What is appropriate technology? What is the relationship between nature and technology? Kluckhohn and Strodtbeck (1961) found three value orientations expressed with regard to this category. Some people value **subjugation to nature**, some value living in **harmony with nature**, and others value **mastery over nature**. Traditionally, mastery over nature has been the dominant orientation of the Old American view, and this value has rationalized the use of any necessary technology to overcome natural forces for the benefit of humans. By extension, an individual has the duty to overcome any obstacle.

Not all Americans have held this orientation. For example, earlier in the 20th century, Kluckhohn and Strodtbeck (1961) found that many Spanish-heritage citizens in the American Southwest reflected a subjugation-to-nature orientation, reflected in a belief that one must adapt to the whims of nature. Many claim that this traditional fatalism finds expression in Spanish aphorisms, such as *Si Díos quiere* ("If God wills it") and *Qué será será* ("Whatever will be, will be"). The value of harmony with nature has been ascribed to Navajo people, as well as to many other cultures, such as the Japanese. Many Navajo rituals involve restoring or establishing a balance between nature and humanity.

Q 2-26. How do you conceptualize the relationship of humans to nature? Do you favor the position that humans should dominate animals and natural resources? What is your reaction to environmental activist groups such as Greenpeace or People for the Ethical Treatment of Animals (PETA)?

2-27. Do you know how you came to hold these values? How do they manifest themselves in your daily life? Are they consistent with the views expressed by your profession?

2-28. How might such views affect the practice of your profession—for example, in dealing with a patient choosing to refuse certain kinds of treatment or to employ alternative treatments?

Time

In its simplest form, the temporal focus of human life can be understood as an emphasis on one dimension—whether past, present, or future. All individuals in all societies must deal with each of these dimensions, but we clearly find preferential orderings among the alternatives. For example, Kluckhohn and Strodtbeck (1961) describe some Hispanics in the Southwest as giving primacy to the present time alternative, paying little attention to what has happened in the past and regarding the future as both vague and unpredictable.

The Aymara, who live in the Andes of Bolivia and Peru, give preference to a past orientation. In fact, in their language they do not have an obligatory tense marker as we do in English to distinguish the present from the past. Instead, they use a marker to distinguish past/present from future. Moreover, like many peoples, the Aymara have a spatial orientation related to time. In English we speak of the future lying in front of us, whereas for the Aymara, the future lies behind, where it cannot be seen because only the past is visible. When the Aymara gesture about time, they gesture ahead of the body to indicate the past and point over their shoulders to refer to the future.

American culture traditionally has placed strong emphasis on the future. This orientation does not mean that we have no concern for the present or past, but that for many of us, considerations of the future tend to dominate our lives. Even when planning for the future is a culturally valued activity, the span of time for which planning is considered reasonable may vary dramatically. American government or business planners typically think in terms of spans of no more than 5 years. Chinese planners, on the other hand, may speak in terms of 50 or 100 years.

2-29. Do you spend more time thinking about the past, the present, or the future? Do you know someone with a different time orientation? How does this person's behavior differ from yours? **Q**

Human Activity

This orientation centers on the nature of self-expression in human activity. Kluckhohn and Strodtbeck (1961) suggest three variations for this conception: being, being-in-becoming, or doing.

In the **being** orientation, the preference is for the kind of activity that is a spontaneous expression of the individual human's essence or **personality**, of impulses and desires. Rowles (1991) notes that a being orientation is essential to individual well-being and argues that it is vital to adopt reflective, self-evaluative approaches to activity.

The **being-in-becoming** orientation also focuses on what the human being is rather than what an individual might accomplish. However, emphasis is on the development of the human essence or personality. "The being-in-becoming orientation emphasizes that kind of activity which has as its goal the development of all aspects of the self as an integrated whole" (Kluckhohn & Strodtbeck, 1961, p. 17).

Traditionally, the **doing** orientation has been the characteristic one in American culture, demanding the kind of activity that results in accomplishments measurable by external standards. Though fulfillment might be an accomplishment of the being-in-becoming orientation, the doing orientation demands accomplishments that can be measured by others: widgets produced, money saved, books written, clients seen.

Q

2-30. Do you think of yourself as having more of a being, becoming, or doing approach to activities? Are some of your valued activities associated with other activity orientations? For example, are you attracted to expressive, impulsive, or reflective leisure activities even though in your work you are driven by an accomplishment orientation?

2-31. In general, what is the activity orientation of your profession? Of the medical system as a whole?

Human Relationships

There are three general ways in which humans relate to each other: lineally, collaterally, and individualistically. These are simply useful analytic concepts because, in reality, all humans relate to others in all three fashions.

All societies recognize the fact that individuals are biologically and culturally related to each other through time; that is, lineally (Kluckhohn & Strodtbeck, 1961). If the lineal orientation is dominant, group goals are dominant, especially the continuity of the group through time. Usually, the lineal principle is expressed through kinship structures.

For example, the English aristocracy is lineal. Irish primogeniture, with the eldest son inheriting the family farm, is another expression of lineality. **Lineality** is a factor in the traditional family form of business, with sons and daughters following their fathers' and mothers' career paths. Fritz Martin (personal communication, 1967) used to tell how he started out sweeping the sawdust on the shop floors. Eventually, he succeeded his father as chairman of the C.F. Martin Company, makers of fine guitars. Martin's career illustrates the lineal principle in the traditional American workplace.

Collaterality is exemplified by sibling relationships. "The individual is not a human being except as... part of a social order, and one type of inevitable social grouping is that which results from laterally extended relationships" (Kluckhohn & Strodtbeck, 1961, p. 18). Collaterality is also the model for the formation of most voluntary associations. Consider, for example, those associations that use fictive kin terminology to define the ideal relationships among members (e.g., lodge "brothers" or sorority "sisters").

Individuality is the third universal relational principle. No society exists where individuals are without autonomy, although in many societies autonomy may be limited. Even though individualism is dominant in America, it is commonly integrated with the other variations of relational orientation. For example, an individualistic American is expected to pursue personal goals of achieving money and prestige in the workplace. At the same time, a worker is expected to subjugate those individualistic goals and assume collateral ones in order to effect teamwork within the organization. If the worker receives a better job offer, however, few would expect that worker not to pursue individualistic goals.

2-32. What values related to human activity and relationships are most important to you? Are these values reflected in the value orientation of your profession? In what ways is your own value orientation similar to the profession's and in what ways does it differ?

Q

These dimensions of universal values interact in both the culture at large and in individuals. Health behaviors and health care also reflect one's general value orientation. That is, your values about health are largely congruent with all of your other values. This congruence is why we can speak of a value *system*. Even though individuals may have very different value systems, almost everyone has a system of well-integrated, congruent values. For example, if individual autonomy is an important value for you, your health care goals may emphasize independence and self-care.

Just as the primary values of an individual may change, so may the collective values of society or some segment of society. Although there are strong forces supporting the continued replication and continuity of values and other cultural components, there also exists the very real chance that significant changes will occur during the transmission process.

CULTURE IS PERSISTENT BUT INCORPORATES CHANGE

Culture changes in two ways. First, the cultural knowledge of an individual continues to change over the life course as he or she encounters new elements in his or her personal environment and incorporates them into his or her life and interactions. As growing numbers of group members adopt such changes, the societal culture begins to change in the second way as well.

At the societal level the collective patterns may change when many individuals alter their customary behaviors. Sometimes such changes occur in a short period of time as a result, for example, of technological innovation or widespread contact with culturally different individuals. Often, cultural change on this level can take several generations.

Cultural Continuity

A defining characteristic of culture is its continuity over time. Thus, change seldom means replacement. Although new cultural components are added to an individual's knowledge base, preexisting components are not excised. Old ideas about technology may be supplanted, but they only cease to exist when they are no longer learned by a new generation. For example, few of us today can shoe a horse or make soap, but we are aware that those used to be common cultural skills.

In his study of Native American myths in South America, Urban (1991) notes how stable myths can be, remaining almost unchanged in the oral tradition for four decades or more. The stability of myths is not guaranteed, however. When there are significant changes in the social environment, these may well be accounted for in myth. Goody and Watt (1963) demonstrated that over a period of 60 years, the myth of origin among the Gonja of northern Ghana changed significantly. When the myth was first recorded around 1900, the myth stated that Ndewura Jakpa came down from the Niger Bend in search of gold, conquered the indigenous inhabitants of the area, enthroned himself as chief of the state, and installed his seven sons as rulers of its territorial divisions. Sixty years later, the myth of origin stated that there were five sons who headed five divisions of the state. What had happened was that during this 60-year period, two of the original divisions were incorporated into a neighboring division, in one case because the ruler had supported a Mandingo invader and in another because of boundary changes introduced by the British administration. Thus, by the 1960s, there were only five clans and the myth very efficiently captured this change.

Goody and Watt (1963) cite this example in a discussion of literacy, noting that when myths are written, especially in sacred books, they may remain stable even thousands of years after they were recorded. The holy books of major religions provide just this sort of stability for believers. Nevertheless, it is clear that when discussing cultural continuity, even in the case of myths, we must recognize that the possibility of change is ever present. For example, current reevaluation of some beliefs about certain American founding fathers is underway as a result of new documents, and even new genetic evidence, as in the case of the descendants of Thomas Jefferson.

Individuals are not only the agents of cultural change but also its mechanism. From early childhood to death, we all acquire new cultural components. Sometimes we add components that are totally new, unlike any other we have previously acquired. Sometimes we acquire components that are similar to ones we already have learned, and these new ones may be in conflict with the old ones. This conflict forces us to evaluate the components and select which one to use, or more rarely, we may combine the two, creatively inventing a third alternative.

A simple example of this process involves changes in food staples. When immigrant families, who are accustomed to a single staple grain or starch in their diets, whether it is rice, corn, or wheat, arrive in the United States, they immediately encounter a wider array of possibilities. How they incorporate these new food items into their own diets, or whether they incorporate them at all, is part of the process of cultural change. Do they keep their traditional grain for special occasions, as does an Italian family we know who serves an elaborate-

THE ENGLISH LANGUAGE AND CULTURAL CHANGE

The original inhabitants of the English Isles were Celtic-speaking peoples whose descendants today speak Gaelic and Welsh, among other languages. The Romans conquered much of what is now England and built a wall in the north to help define their southern territory. In addition to Hadrian's Wall and public baths, the Romans also left some Latin behind, incorporated into Celtic, when they retreated to Rome. Some time later, in 453, a group of Anglo-Saxon mercenaries arrived from Germany to help some native Celts defend their homeland from Norse-speaking Viking invaders. The Anglos and the Saxons spoke an early form of German, which was laid over the pre-existing Celtic/Latin language mix. Then, in 1066, French-speaking Normans conquered the English Isles and imposed French, a much altered form of Latin, as the language of government.

Thus, English actually began as a mid-fifth century kind of German, built on a base of Celtic and Latin. The massive influx of French altered it substantially, vastly expanding the vocabulary. Dual sets of references abounded, such as the use of Anglo-Saxon words, like *cow*, to refer to an animal, and French words, like *beef*, to refer to its food form. Because of its relation to Latin, French also increased the amount of Latinate vocabulary, producing many pairs of synonymous words, one Germanic in origin and the other Latinate, such as *shape* and *form*. New sounds were also added to the language during this period, such as the sound represented by the letters *ge* in *rouge*, itself a French word for *red*.

Later, during the colonial period, indigenous peoples from around the British empire contributed words, as well as sounds, meanings, and structures from their native languages, to form the regional dialects we hear in the speech of Americans, Indians, Jamaicans, Kenyans, and others. Of course, even without culture contact as a source of language change, the English language would not have remained stable. Even before the Normans arrived, the German varieties spoken on the continent and that spoken in the English Isles were no longer mutually intelligible. The English, as they are now called, invented their own new words and linguistic forms.

The story does not end there. After achieving independence, the language in at least one former colony changed considerably. In the United States, immigrants from other countries have added myriad new words and expressions to American English. Each generation creates its own additions to the language as well, in an evolving process that continues to this day.

---

ly prepared spaghetti as its Thanksgiving dinner centerpiece? Do they standardize combinations of new and old foods, as when a Burmese family serves rice with vegetable meals but incorporates bread and potatoes with grilled meats? The success of many restaurants has been built on the fusion of cuisine types, such as Caribbean and Thai in single menu items.

Q 2-33. Think about your own favorite foods and note a few of them in the margin. How many of them are traditional for your ethnic or cultural community?

2-34. Make a list of some of the new food ingredients you have sampled within the last 5 years. Where did each item come from? How have you incorporated the items into your diet? How many different cultural groups are reflected in your meal planning and preparation?

Obviously, the introduction of new food items is a fairly simple example of culture change, which is a complex and long-term process. It affects value orientations, social organization, human relationships, and economic behaviors, along with many other aspects of culture. Whatever we do when we face new alternatives is significant in terms of the process of social change. We either perpetuate the traditional or tempt change by the choices we make. The collection of all such actions by the members of a society dictates the cultural future of the entire society.

The Process of Culture Change

Wallace (1970) was among the first social scientists to insist that in order to understand how groups of very different individuals organize themselves into orderly, adaptive, changing societies, we must study the cognitive processes of many individuals. Culture is never constant because the individuals in a society are always adapting to their ever-changing environments. Some cultures may be subjected to more rapid change than others at any moment in time, as were the Hmong as a result of their military alliance with the United States. Some cultures seem more resistant to external forces. Hopi religion is widely acknowledged to be almost unchanged even after 500 years of missionary work and evangelization.

Change may affect one part of society more rapidly than another, as was the case when barbed wire was introduced into the American West. When farmers began to populate the West and fenced their property with this new-fangled invention, they precipitated change in the rancher culture, which was accustomed to, and highly valued, the concept of the "free range." The dislocation produced during this contest over principles of land ownership and use, individual autonomy, and economic impact even led to violence in some cases. The direct impact of this conflict of values was not much felt in the urbanized East. However, the cultural change that subordinated cattle drives to agriculture resonated decades later in popular culture artifacts such as film and cowboy songs that were enjoyed across the country. It still lives on in today's political wrangling over federal land use and the values incorporated in the food term "free range chicken."

Change can also be sudden, through the effects of war or epidemic. Many societies today are experiencing drastic culture change from such factors as technological innovation, immigration, changes in political processes, forced relocation, epidemics, famines, and war. The presence of human immunodeficiency virus (HIV) infection in some parts of Africa is now at such an elevated level that it is likely to provoke catastrophic social change in a very short time.

Because language and culture are so closely intertwined, we can often see evidence of culture change in the ways that language changes over time. New inventions require new words (e.g., "airplane") and contact among cultures can lead to sharing of words (e.g., "salsa"). The English language provides a good example of the way in which a language incorporates into its grammar and vocabulary the effects of cultural contact and change. Consider a brief history of English provided in the box on page 38.

Q 2-35. Think about your own experience with English. What words do you use that you can identify as coming from other languages, such as Spanish, Yiddish, or French? List a few of them in the margins, indicating their probable language of origin.

2-36. What words do you know that are associated with specific generations?

Cultures may also change through innovation or acculturation. **Innovation** may take the form of a technological invention or new ideas about how to do things. **Acculturation** is the process of borrowing ideas, things, or processes from another culture. For example, immigrants to the United States from developing countries will, over time, accommodate to the differences in health care. They will learn, among other things, that in order to obtain the antibiotics they got at home simply by going to the pharmacy, they must now first visit a physician who will provide a prescription. Once a new element has diffused through a culture, it may be said to be a general component of the culture because it is widely shared.

Groups can deliberately alter the life patterns of individuals through rites of passage. Similarly, individuals' life patterns can be affected by drastic changes in environmental conditions. Under either situation, an individual may develop new goals, values, tactics, or relationships that reflect the process of culture emergent (Clifton, 1976).

All life involves change. There is evolutionary change as species, including *Homo sapiens*, adapt to the environment over time. There is individual change as living organisms grow through the life stages. An individual person matures from birth until death stops the process. All these changes involve social as well as biological developments. There is also cultural change as communities of people adapt to the conditions of their local environment through different technologies, behaviors, and beliefs. There can be no individual who does not change. Thus, enculturation continues throughout life. No one ever learns all there is to know about his or her culture. Likewise, there can be no culture that does not change. Therefore, cultural values, beliefs, and norms are in a constant state of evolution.

Predicting change for an individual or for many individuals within a society is difficult. Understanding the change process—how some things change rapidly at a given moment or under specific circumstances while other things change much more slowly and how such changes are managed culturally—may be the most critical element in understanding the human condition.

CONCEPTS OF RACE AND ETHNICITY

We must note here that culture is not equivalent to race or ethnicity. These two constructs are sometimes used as proxies for cultural identification, but both are limited or problematic in significant ways.

Race, like culture, is difficult to define. It is often thought of as an inherited (i.e., biological) trait that can be seen in physical appearance. However, making racial distinctions on the basis of appearance is risky. Consider the many light-skinned African-Americans living in the United States or the blonde, blue-eyed individuals living near the Mediterranean Sea. Recent genetic findings (Angier, 2000) suggest that the differences in DNA between so-called racial groups are minuscule, causing many scientists to assert that the concept of race simply has no valid biological basis. Even though we can identify specific groups that carry different risks for some diseases (e.g., sickle cell anemia among persons of African descent [Masi & Disman, 1994]) this pattern is probably a function of generations of reproduction by individuals in close geographic proximity, rather than some inherent "racial" factor.

That said, there is no question that in many cultures, distinctions are made among groups with differing physical characteristics. Sephardic Jews, those of Mediterranean descent, are thought to be typically swarthy or olive-skinned, with dark hair and eyes and prominent noses, a description that obviously fits many other groups as well. In Israel, individuals with these traits are considered to have lower status than Ashkenazi (European) Jews, with their light hair and blue eyes. In Scandinavia, Swedes distinguish their Norwegian cousins (with "dark" hair) from those from Iceland (with very blonde hair). In the United States, racial distinctions have had profound social and economic consequences for centuries (Malcomson, 2000). We do not dispute the power of race as a social construct, particularly among European-derived cultures; however, we consider race to be inadequate as an alternative for the concept of culture.

Ethnicity is also somewhat tricky as a proxy for culture. **Ethnicity** is typically used to identify presumed (or most readily identifiable) country of origin, such as Italian or Polish. In the United States, ethnicity is often combined with "American"; for example, Italian-American. The problem with ethnicity as a stand-in for culture has to do in part with our faulty memories and historical awareness. One of the authors of this book was raised to believe that she was Russian-American. On the dissolution of the Union of Soviet Socialist Republics, she was startled to discover that she actually came from what was now identified as a separate country, Ukraine. More recently, she learned that the part of Ukraine from which her family emigrated had long ago been invaded by Norwegians, perhaps explaining her blue eyes. Thus, her firmly held ethnic identity has repeatedly been called into question.

Further, few people in the United States can now trace their ethnic origin to a single group. As immigration, intermarriage, and acculturation have proceeded, the number of descriptors in a single individual's identity has increased while temporal distance from ethnic origin has grown. The children of the Russian-Ukrainian-Norwegian-American woman must add their father's English, French, Native American, Irish, and Scots ancestry to their list. In any case, none of these ethnic components is foremost in the self identities of her children.

2-37. What do you describe as your racial identity? How do you think this identity relates to your cultural values and beliefs? **Q**

2-38. What is your description of your ethnicity? How closely do you think your behaviors and beliefs reflect the country of origin for that ethnicity?

The next chapter considers how individual personality and learning interacts with cultural factors to create unique cultural interpretations, a culture emergent, for each individual.

✎ NOTES ✎

✎ Notes ✐

CHAPTER

3

Personality and Culture

CHAPTER OBJECTIVES

By the end of this chapter, the reader will be able to:

1. Distinguish between individual personality and biological factors and the influence of culture.
2. Discuss the impact of biological (genetic, physiologic) forces on behavior.
3. List and describe individual factors relevant to personality development.
4. List and describe cultural factors relevant to personality development.
5. Discuss the interaction of personal and cultural factors in personality development.
6. Describe the ways in which culture influences behavior.
7. Describe the ways in which individuals enact personal characteristics within cultural constraints.
8. Discuss issues of multiculturalism and the effects of multicultural societies on individual behavior.
9. Describe the value of cultural stereotypes.
10. Describe the dilemmas presented by cultural stereotypes.
11. Describe the ways in which contact among individuals affects culture change.

THE STORY OF LIA LEE

In the last chapter, we briefly described some features of Hmong culture and explained how the Lees were brought into contact with Western medicine. Here we provide additional history, with particular emphasis on the interaction of Hmong culture with the personalities and life circumstances of Nao Kao Lee, Foua, and their daughter Lia Lee.

Following Hmong tradition, Foua was encouraged to respond to her food cravings during pregnancy, as failure to do so could have resulted in a blemish on the child. Nao Kao could bring her water during delivery only if he did not look at her; it is considered inappropriate for a husband to see his wife's body during labor. Foua was expected to be silent during labor, but in the hospital she did not squat on the floor and catch her baby herself, nor did Nao Kao cut the umbilical cord. Because there were no problems during labor, traditional remedies were not required, and, in any case, the hospital would not have permitted them.

At birth, Lia Lee weighed 8 pounds, 7 ounces. Lia was to all appearances healthy, and she received Apgar scores of 7 and 9. However, her birth was quite different from a typical Hmong birth; she was the first of her siblings born in a hospital, with physicians in attendance. Her mother did not take the placenta home and bury it in the house to help the soul travel back to its roots, as Hmong custom dictated. The physicians did not understand the custom; some thought that the Hmong ate the placentas.

After his wife gave birth, Nao Kao brought Foua a special chicken soup believed to be the only safe thing to eat during the next 30 days, along with rice. The health care providers in Merced reacted to this behavior in different ways. One said, "The Hmong men carried these nice little silver cans to the hospital that always had some kind of chicken soup in them and always smelled great." Another said, "They always brought some horrible stinking concoction that smelled like the chicken had been dead for a week" (Fadiman, 1997, p. 9).

A naming ceremony, a soul-calling, took place when Lia was about a month old (in Laos it would have been celebrated on the third day after birth, the time at which an infant is considered fully human by the Hmong). Lia's ceremony, in the family's apartment, involved the sacrifice of a pig and two chickens, which were examined for signs concerning the name to be chosen for the infant. Then all the food was cooked and consumed by the guests. Lia was brushed with a bundle of white strings to sweep away illness, and a string was tied around each wrist to bind her soul to her body. In addition to the strings, the Lees gave Lia a number of decorative hats to make her look like a flower from above, where the *dabs* (evil spirits) would be looking down for vulnerable children. She was given a silver necklace with a soul-retaining lock and was carried in a cloth with a soul-retaining design.

The Lees clung to these traditions, reluctant to let go of their history. They felt uncomfortable in the United States. The situation was perhaps worst for Nao Kao, because the structure of his life was more disrupted. He no longer had his agricultural work, nor his role and status in the community. Foua still had a home to manage and children to look after, giving her at least a semblance of her previous situation. The Lees missed their previous life but recognized that they had greater financial stability in the United States. In addition, when Lia had her first seizure, they felt that the United States medical system, something not previously available to them, might help.

Summarized from Fadiman, A. (1997). *The spirit catches you and you fall down*. New York: Noonday Press.

INTRODUCTION

We have established that culture is shared, is learned, and has meaning. We have also established that culture is emergent in the patterned interactions and behaviors of individuals and that it is subject to change. However, behavior is shaped by more than culture. Individual personality and biology strongly influence how an individual will share cultural values, what the individual will learn, and the meaning of the culture for that individual. Thus, there is an interplay between culture and individual personality, biology, and experience, as well as among the various cultural groups to which every individual unavoidably belongs. At the same time, culture is constantly changing, emergent not only in the experiences of individuals in the culture, but also responsive to changes in the social, physical, and political environment. The result of this complex interaction of factors is each person's development of an idiosyncratic set of beliefs and behaviors evident in his or her daily life. As it is important to understand culture, it is equally important to understand individual development. Further, it is vital to recognize the interaction of all these factors in order to facilitate genuine understanding of the individual within the context of culture.

The complexity of these relationships makes it clear that knowledge of an individual's cultural background may provide some information about personal characteristics, but it is unlikely that knowledge of that single factor will adequately describe the person. Because biological, personality, and cultural factors interact in individual experience and because individuals express only some facets of their complex identities in any single interaction, understanding everything potentially significant about a patient or client is impossible. However, the concept of culture emergent can help clinicians become more aware of these interacting factors and how they affect health care. In this chapter, we explore the interactions of culture with biological and personal characteristics, and the relative influence of these factors on values and behaviors.

PERSONALITY AND CULTURE

Some definitions of culture leave out the reality of individual difference. "The very focus on differences between cultures has led to an emphasis on homogeneity within cultures" (Wainryb, 1997, p. 52). These definitions typically describe cultural rules as relatively set, universally shared values that lead to predictable behaviors by individuals within the culture. When an outsider observes a culture, her or his first impressions may be of the most typical behaviors rather than the full spectrum actually present. These first impressions form the basis of general descriptions. For example, if you were to travel to Paris, never having been there before, you might describe the culture in terms of beautiful architecture, wonderful food, and haughty people. Initial impressions change over time. If your first effort to communicate in French is met with smiles and encouragement, your perception of the French as haughty might be immediately altered. In the same way, initial impressions of clients reflect the most readily observed characteristics (single, white, well-nourished, middle-aged woman, for example). As we move beyond outsider status and acquire additional information, descriptions become richer and probably more accurate, reflecting a broader gamut of variability that reflects the individual as a member of the group but not synonymous with it. The "single, white, well-nourished, middle-aged woman," for instance, may be an enthusiastic supporter of feminism or the National Rifle Association (or both), may be assertive or shy, may be ambitious or laid-back.

Some theorists have posited that the "self" as an individual is a Western construction (Geertz, 1984). These theorists suggest that culture dictates individual behavior and interpersonal interaction. Nucci (1997) calls such theorists **social constructivists** who seem to "embrace a psychological relativism in which personhood and the individual are cultural variants rather than expressions of some underlying set of psychological realities" (p. 6). This view suggests that the self does not actually exist, but rather that individuals exist as representatives or reflections of their culture. In this view, individual variability would be assumed to be relatively minimal. Other theorists believe that

> conceptions of self as distinct and particular are linked to the existence of arenas of personal choice, and that choice appears as a cross-cultural universal precisely because it is a psychological requirement for the construction of distinct and bounded selves. (Nucci, 1997, p. 6)

In other words, the establishment of a self as distinct from the group requires some element of choice, and some degree of choice must therefore exist in every culture. Though the choice may be circumscribed in some cultures, individuality still emerges. Even such choices as how to make a tradi-

Figure 3-1. This Mayan woman uses a low stool to weave on the backstrap loom. Note the generally low height for other tables and chairs in the space.

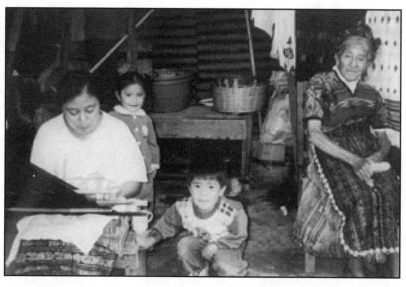

tional dish (should the matzo balls be light or heavy?) reflect the individual and his or her tastes. When Mayan women engage in backstrap weaving (Figure 3-1), some sit on low stools or sit quite still on traditional palm leaf mats; others frequently shift position. These differences may be matters of personal choice or family tradition but are not culturally prescribed even though the form for backstrap weaving is very much a cultural tradition.

Q

3-1. Think of an activity that you and almost everyone in your family or religious group or set of friends performs regularly. Examples might be studying or writing, celebrating an annual holiday, or grocery shopping. In the margins, note the commonalities you share while engaging in this activity. Then note the differences. To an outsider, would you all look as if you were doing the "same thing"?

3-2. Think of an activity in which you and your professional colleagues engage routinely. Answer the same set of questions.

As noted in Chapter 2, every culture has a status structure in which there are ascribed and achieved statuses. Both kinds of status interact with individual propensities, sometimes reflecting a good match, other times causing difficulty for the individual. For example, among British royalty, status is rigidly ascribed. The firstborn son of the ruling monarch is destined to be king regardless of personality. The history of the British monarchy vividly demonstrates that this ascribed status is enacted very differently depending on the individual, sometimes with excellent outcomes, sometimes with disaster when a crown prince (or, in a few cases, princess) is poorly suited to the role. Daughters or second sons who might make better rulers must instead adjust to other expectations.

Status is enacted through the fulfillment of roles, but individual propensities strongly influence the way in which those roles will be enacted. Consider the women you know who are mothers. Each puts her own unique mark on the role. Some might focus on emotional nurturing, others on inculcating their children with particular values. Some might interact primarily around craft projects while others teach their children to bake or to camp. Thus, although the social role carries a single name, it strongly reflects the unique characteristics and interests of the individual.

The process of identity formation requires the merging of group and individual identities (Belay, 1996). Ideally, these merge into a coherent self. "Individuals within cultures participate in multifaceted social experiences and in the process develop distinct goals, interests, and perspectives" (Wainryb, 1997, p. 32). Even in highly communal cultures where group goals and cooperation are emphasized, some individuals will tend to be outspoken; others, more reticent. These individual characteristics, whether biological or learned, if widely distributed, can affect the cultural development of the society. For example, at the present time in Japan, a significant number of young women are choosing to remain unmarried because their personal wishes do not fit the cultural expectations about the behavior of a "good" wife. Rather than try to obviate the personal, they reject cultural norms.

Q 3-3. Can you think of an area of life in which you have defied or subverted cultural norms? What motivated you to do so? Have you experienced any conflict as a result? Do you know of other people who have made similar choices on similar grounds?

Bandlamudi (1994) suggests that there is great complexity in the ways in which individuals locate themselves in the cultural matrix. In a study of multiethnic adolescents in New York, he examined the ways in which participants described themselves as fitting into the culture. Five categories emerged, each chosen by a subset of the participants. The categories range from one he labels nonrelational subjectivism/objectivism, in which the self is perceived as completely differentiated from the culture and defined solely in terms of unique personal traits, to the dialogical/dialectical category, in which the distinction between self and culture breaks down, creating a constant state of tension and resulting in change for both individuals and cultures. This research makes clear that adolescents recognize that they exist as unique individuals but also that they exist in the context of culture.

Personality, a reflection of the self, is "an individual's characteristic pattern of thought, emotion, and behavior, together with the psychological mechanisms—hidden or not—behind those patterns" (Funder, 1997, pp. 1–2). Personality development occurs through the interplay of individual and sociocultural factors, as limited or expanded by structural or material constraints (Miller, 1997). Evidence from an array of studies of culture suggests that the self exists in every culture and that unique individual characteristics can be identified regardless of the extent to which the culture may be described as **collectivist**, or focused on group goals (i.e., communally oriented).

BIOLOGY AND BEHAVIOR

Biological inheritance influences human behavior (Massimini & Fave, 2000). Biological predispositions are based on genetic factors and prenatal influences on development. Skin color, body shape and size, and hair color and texture are all genetically determined and have a direct relation to

ascribed membership in culturally-specified groups. It is equally true that some behavioral predispositions are also genetic. Parents describe differences among their offspring as evident from the day of birth. One child may be quiet, observant, and introspective, another active and outgoing. Such differences can be observed well before parental, situational, or cultural factors could have influenced them and may persist throughout life. Similarly, prenatal influences may alter behavior before the external environment can have an impact. The most striking examples include the impact of prenatal exposure to teratogenic drugs (e.g., alcohol); it is equally likely that other factors such as maternal stress, nutrition, and hormone levels can also affect the temperament of the newborn. Parents recognize that their own reactions to their children, and their behaviors with them, are influenced not only by the gender of the child but also by some of these innate personality characteristics of the child. It is typical within many cultural groups to hear parents describe their infants as "sweet," "placid," or "active," and as "easier than her brother," "a real character," and so on.

There has been considerable recent research examining contributions of biology to behavior and belief, and a consensus is emerging that biological factors are much more salient than previously believed. Such behaviors as altruism may have a biological foundation (Low, 1999) and appear to play an important role in preservation of the species. Animal studies suggest that altruism is important to preservation of species as opposed to survival of individuals; thus it plays an important evolutionary function.

The study of gender differences has been particularly intriguing in examining the biological substrates of behavior (Blum, 1997; Colapinto, 2000; Low, 1999). Gender differences in brain function provide possible biological explanations for some differential gender behaviors and perceptions. For example, the now well-known delineation of "right brain" (creative, feminine) versus "left brain" (analytic, male) originated with studies focused on gender difference in cortical function. Such differences may be the result of genetic influences or other biological factors, such as prenatal exposure to hormones.

Cases of gender assignment where gender is not easily observed provide clear evidence that **gender identity** (one's sense of being male or female) is formed very early, well before social influences can affect it. Colapinto (2000) reports the case of Joan/John, one of a number of infants who, during the 1960s and 1970s, were patients of Dr. J. Money. When John was an infant, his penis was accidentally cut off. Money recommended that he be reassigned as female, and John's testes were removed. At puberty, hormone therapy was instituted to promote female development. Nevertheless, when Joan reached adolescence, she was profoundly unhappy. When she discovered her history and reassumed her male identity, she found herself much more satisfied and content. It is unclear whether it was the presence of the Y chromosome or prenatal exposure to particular levels of testosterone that led to John's male gender identity. In either case, however, that identification was sufficiently imprinted by birth to obviate multiple, massive efforts at reassignment from birth to adolescence.

Understanding of the precise nature of gender difference is emerging gradually. Initial studies early in the century suggested profound differences (as reflected, for example, in Freud's writings), whereas in the 1960s differences were disputed. Feminist theorists suggested that the differences were a matter of enculturation, not biology. More recent work challenges the dogmatism of this idea. It is increasingly clear that there are biological differences between women and men that may influence behavior in significant ways. Even so, much gender-marked behavior is the consequence of culturally defined patterns overlaid on this biological base. As elsewhere, biology and culture interact.

Some biological studies present intriguing questions regarding the understanding of the relationship between individuals and cultural difference. Studies of twins separated at birth and raised in different environments show that behavioral characteristics are deeply embedded biologically (Wright, 1997). Such twins show similar levels of intelligence, personality characteristics, and even behavioral quirks such as fingernail biting or hair twirling. Even for twins, however, environmental factors are important (Collins et al., 2000). Some studies of twins separated at birth have shown that those taken from dysfunctional homes and raised by more effective families are much less likely to demonstrate dysfunctional behaviors than those raised in the family of origin.

Likewise, some attributes that might be considered biological show profound cultural difference. For example, there is evidence that individuals raised in Chinese culture have superior visual processing skills as compared with individuals in the United States (Yoon et al., 2000). The same research showed that individuals with hearing impairments who learned American sign language also have superior visual processing skills. The researchers speculate that the difference can be attributed to use of ideographic language systems as opposed to any inherent biological difference among these groups. Peng and Nisbett (1999) found similar differences in preferred reasoning strategies between individuals in the United States and China, and attribute these differences to culturally mediated strategies for learning.

There is a good bit of controversy about the relative contributions of biology and culture to human behavior (M. Goode, 2000). Recent genetic studies suggest that in spite of the apparent major differences among people, the ancestry of all humanity can be traced to 10 men and 18 women (Wade, 2000). There is obvious concern about the potential to reduce humanity to a collection of genes, and clearly the astounding differences among people must result from something besides genetic inheritance. The mixing and matching of the genetic material of even only 18 individuals produces such an array of possible combinations that it is impossible to sort out just what is the specific genetic inheritance. Rather, biological inheritance must be put in the context of the multiple influences on human development. Biology alone has failed to explain human behavior fully (Horgan, 1996). Although the contribution of biology to behavior cannot be ignored, we must look further to understand individual variation (Figure 3-2).

3-4. Examine your own beliefs about the role of biology on human behavior. Do you think it plays a big role or is it not very important? How would you summarize your position on this controversial issue?

3-5. What evidence has led you to hold this position? Does your opinion affect your professional relations?

INDIVIDUAL FACTORS IN PERSONALITY DEVELOPMENT

There are myriad theories of personality development (Funder, 1997), most of which acknowledge the realities of biology. They posit that in addition to genetics, an array of pre- and post-natal mechanisms further influence the development of personality traits. Such mechanisms include birth order, parental influence, learning, environmental conditions, and so on. Most of these theories have

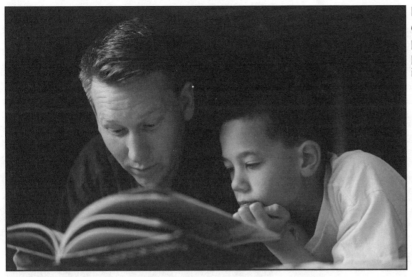

Figure 3-2. Adopted children whose physical appearance differs from their parents' will still be raised in the parents' culture.

been developed with a focus on Western societies; there is less understanding about personality development in other cultures. However, there is clear evidence that even in the most **communitarian** of cultures, individual traits and personalities are evident. Individuals do not all look the same despite their common physical traits, nor do they all behave and feel the same despite whatever common experiences they may have. Nucci (1997) indicates that in every culture, a sphere of behavior that is to some extent personal inevitably emerges. Foua and Nao Kao Lee, Lia Lee's parents, had different reactions to their move to the United States. Nao Kao found the adjustment more difficult (Fadiman, 1997). Though environmental factors such as the loss of his role as provider for his family may have played a role in this difficulty, it is likely that personality factors were also involved, as some other Hmong men might have found the move less problematic than did Nao Kao.

Consider the example of two sisters born to an alcoholic father. The father's behavior was unpredictable, dependent on whether and how much alcohol he had consumed. Both sisters lived with this unpredictability throughout their childhood, until the day their father left home. At that time, one sister was age 11, the other 13. One of the sisters had, by that time, solved the problem of family strife by becoming involved in an array of outside activities. She belonged to the school band, practicing every day after school. She participated in a church youth group that took many weekend trips away from the city. Her teachers and youth group leaders, aware of her situation and impressed by her courage, took her under their wing and served as

surrogate parents for her, providing the support and encouragement she greatly needed. The younger sister, shy by nature and intimidated by her father, did not create such alternatives for herself. She worried about her parents, trying hard to convince her father to quit drinking, and to help her mother cope. As time went on, she became more withdrawn, quiet, and isolated. These two girls shared the same home environment, but personal and situational characteristics led them to experience the environment in different ways.

A basic requirement for psychological integrity includes establishment of an arena of personal choice and privacy. There is no question that the realm of personal choice and the amount of privacy available varies depending upon cultural norms. Even in communitarian cultures, however, people have different roles, positions, and experiences in their families, daily events, and personal reactions and emotions (Funder, 1997).

Regardless of the boundaries of the personal, psychological interpretation occurs twice: on the societal level (between people) and on the individual level (Vygotsky, 1978). As events unfold, interpersonal processes are transformed into intrapersonal ones and vice versa. Take the example of ritual, an important element of culture. All social rituals have both inter- and intrapersonal aspects. The interpersonal aspects of ritual emphasize the patterned ways in which the ritual guides interaction with others. For instance, religious services all have a format by which people share the experience of worship. That structure varies widely from, for example, a Quaker meeting to a Catholic mass; but within each group, a particular pattern of interaction with others is specified. At the same time, each individual has her or his own experience of the worship. A personal meaning is taken from what is largely a communal activity.

Q   3-6.   Think back to the regular activity you considered earlier in question 3-1, in which you and a group of people all participate together. What are your feelings as you participate? How would you characterize the personal meaning the activity has for you? Do you think the others who also engage in it share the feelings and meanings you experience?

CULTURAL FACTORS IN PERSONALITY DEVELOPMENT

Culture—the shared, learned values and beliefs that structure meaning—has its own influence on personality development. "Selves are always culturally and temporally situated" (Nucci, 1997, p. 6). Individual characteristics are molded by the surrounding environment, such that an individual who is temperamentally inclined toward ebullience may, in some cultures, express this trait in relatively muted fashion. In traditional Chinese culture, for example, displays of strong emotion are not considered appropriate; young children are taught to be subdued and to mask their feelings. However, some Chinese children are more expressive than others.

In the United States, there is a tendency to be highly expressive of emotions, although there are many children who are shy and reticent.

Nucci (1997) suggests that cultural molding of child behavior is accomplished initially through parental influence. During childhood, personal choice is relatively circumscribed, with parents having significant influence on moral and behavioral expectations. Parental responsibility for regulation of moral conduct continues into adolescence, while the sphere of behavior considered personal expands. Domains of autonomy are culturally variable (Miller, 1997) so that what is considered personal in one culture (choice of a spouse or a career, for example) might be considered a family or societal responsibility in another. Where personal choice is more circumscribed, individuality may be expressed more subtly. A young woman living in a culture where arranged marriage is the norm may resort to subtle demonstration that she is not happy with her family's choice for her rather than to direct rebellion against tradition.

INTERACTION OF THE PERSONAL AND THE CULTURAL

Ultimately, behavior is mediated by both personal and cultural factors. Consider the behavior of

CULTURE AND PERSONALITY IN CAREER CHOICE

There is a significant body of literature suggesting that people make career choices based on the match between their personalities and the expectations of the professional culture (Spokane, 1992; Tokar, Fischer, & Subich, 1998). Further, within a particular profession, specialty choices are based on personality factors and personal values (Hoff, 1998; Hojat et al., 1998; Lewicki et al., 1999). This sorting process appears to occur as students become more familiar with the profession for which they are training and make choices that further refine the match between their personal characteristics and the specialty areas. For example, for occupational therapy students, culminating fieldwork experiences strongly influence choice of practice area, a reflection of an individual's personal comfort with a particular professional environment or culture. Additional factors that enter the equation for career choice include gender and developmental life stage (Craik & Alderman, 1998; DeVoe, Kennedy, & Pena, 1998).

Career choice reflects the characteristics of particular professions, and the attraction of particular kinds of individuals to those professions reinforces the nature of the professions. For example, Mattingly (1998) notes that "occupational therapists say, 'Nurses do for patients. We help patients do for themselves'" (p. 74). Although one may not agree with the specific content of this delineation, it reflects a recognition that professions have their own values and beliefs (i.e., that they are cultures).

adult children toward their aging parents. Such interactions are inevitably colored by personality characteristics and personal experience. One adult child may avoid parents because of childhood perceptions of rejection; his or her sibling may be deeply involved with the parents. At the same time, cultural factors also enter into behavioral patterns. For example, in India, cultural values foster a sense of obligation to help others (Miller & Bersoff, 1992). This sense of obligation typically leads adult children to take care of their aging parents and to support them both financially and instrumentally. As in Western culture, however, some will do more than others, moving in with parents or visiting every day, while siblings visit only weekly.

In Herero culture in southern Africa, elders are viewed as keepers of cultural wisdom (Draper & Harpending, 1994). They adopt a largely ceremonial role and are assisted in their daily tasks by younger individuals. Here, too, not all adult children are equally willing to provide for their elders. Long-standing interpersonal conflict, differences in personal perception, and differences in individual situation may all affect the extent to which adults enact this cultural value.

These examples demonstrate the ways in which cultural values are affected by personal characteristics. In both Indian and Herero cultures, there is an explicit value that states that adult children should respect and care for their aging parents. In both cultures, there are strong societal messages reflecting this value; that is, there are significant pressures toward enculturation of the child with the value. Individual personality, however, has an impact on the extent to which each adult child will conform to the behavior dictated by that value. Many fundamental human choices (e.g., the choice of career) reflect an interaction among individual personality characteristics, the cultural values enculturated by the family, and the cultural characteristics of the career or profession, as well as environmental factors relating to exposure, access, and social value.

Q

3-7. Think about your own profession as a culture. Jot down some of the characteristics of this culture.

3-8. Now think about the kinds of people who are attracted to your profession. Jot down a list of personal characteristics that you believe to be typical of your profession.

3-9. Now think about yourself. How well do your characteristics match those you believe typical of individuals in your profession? In what ways do you match the description? In what ways are you different?

3-10. If possible, share your list with someone in the same profession. Do your descriptions match hers or his? How are they similar? How are they different?

A complicating factor in the development of the individual is the fact that in complex societies he or she inevitably belongs to multiple cultures (Belay, 1996). Among the cultures to which the individual belongs are religious, ethnic, occupational, and national groups. All are nonuniform and impermanent, providing yet another source of variability in individual experience. An Indian friend described how conflicted she felt about her aging parents back home; although she was able to live up to some of her obligations by sending money to them, she was unavailable to provide instrumental support. However, she had also incorporated some Western beliefs and felt that she needed to put herself and her own children first, rather than move back to India as her parents' health deteriorated. She also felt that her work as a psychologist gave her additional responsibility to her patients rather than just to her family. She was caught in conflicts of roles and values set up by her participation in multiple cultures.

It is therefore important to recognize that the nature of the person is not fixed by birth but evolves over time. Although many characteristics have a biological basis, new experiences have an impact on the expression of those characteristics. Each time an individual enters a new group or shifts among groups, his or her behaviors, values, and attitudes may shift. Because there is no such thing as **cultural exclusivity**—the existence of a single culture in the absence of all others—it is vital to attend to the importance of the processes of acculturation and adaptation as these influence identity development. For example, there have been recent reports on the incorporation of the Internet into Central American cultures, opening a window to other parts of the world previously inaccessible to them (Ellin, 2000). Such interaction will inevitably change Central American cultures; just adding the word "Internet" to Spanish represents a minor cultural modification.

The Force of Culture on the Individual

No doubt you have followed the stories emerging from Afghanistan about the dramatic changes in the status of women since the Taliban took control of the government. The Taliban, run by fundamentalist Muslim men, incorporates a strict interpretation of Muslim rules about women's behavior. In fact, the Taliban has gone beyond those rules, insisting that women go outside their homes only if accompanied by an adult male family member and covered head to foot in robes. Even the face must be completely covered. Women have not been able to hold employment outside the home, and receive no education. Under Taliban control, women trained as physicians and teachers could no longer practice their professions. Among the many serious consequences of these edicts is the absence of medical care for women, since in this culture men cannot serve as physicians for women.

Despite these strictures, some women have found ways to protest the restrictions, leading to international condemnation of the Taliban by women's rights activists. Individual women have risked death making efforts to get information out of Afghanistan to pressure the government for change. Culture has a profound impact on these women; however, their personal characteristics still modify their actions. Not all women choose to protest—it is a matter of individual personality and values, the product of a unique combination of biology, environment, context, and experience.

Cultural norms place particular expectations on individuals and sanctions those who do not meet expectations. The huge market for self-help books in the United States is, in part, a reflection of people's perceived failure in living up to those expectations or their desire to escape them. In the United States, the dominant culture is one in which we expect people to be physically attractive, preferably young and athletic, upwardly mobile, involved in a permanent relationship with someone of the opposite sex, and happy. People who wander too far from that set of expectations often experience a sense of disapproval from those around them. For example, in some groups, once a couple has married (ideally in their early to mid-20s), it is considered fair to inquire about their plans for children and to note with surprise and disapproval their failure to produce progeny within a reasonable time. Similarly, middle-aged men are expected to move from job to job up a ladder toward increasing responsibility and reward. Those who do not conform to these expec-tations may perceive themselves as failures and sometimes receive messages from others to support that perception. It is worth noting that these expectations can remain relatively stable in a given culture but may or may not reflect the actual behavior of the majority of people.

Although the values described above reflect the dominant culture in the United States, there are many competing cultural groups that have their own prescriptive norms for behavior. Among some groups, children may come before or without marriage. In others, marriage may come first but at a relatively older age. In some groups, male unemployment may be so common as to be unremarkable. Any of these situations may be beyond an individual's control.

Individual Variation Within Cultures

Although culture prescribes particular sets of values and beliefs, these are strongly mediated by individual characteristics such as education, breadth of experience, living situation, and a multitude of other factors. Recall, for example, your most recent Thanksgiving holiday. In the United States, Thanksgiving has particular cultural meaning and expression; it is an important cultural ritual. A typical Thanksgiving involves a celebratory meal. If the media are to be believed, that meal includes turkey, cranberry relish, and a huge, happy, and neatly attired family. Perhaps a game of touch football follows the meal, and almost certainly some time is spent watching sports on television.

Your own Thanksgiving may have diverged from that model in significant ways. Perhaps you do not have a large family or perhaps they are too far away to enable you to spend the day with them. Perhaps you are a vegetarian who dined on tofu rather than turkey; there is tremendous cultural variation with regard to celebratory foods. Perhaps you offered to work that day so that some of your coworkers with small children would not have to. Perhaps you served Thanksgiving dinners at a homeless shelter. It may be that there are interpersonal tensions in your family or maybe it was the first Thanksgiving following the death of someone central to the family. Any of these factors might result in a Thanksgiving that differs from the popularized ideal.

As further evidence of the importance of individual personality as a mediating factor in interpreting culture, think about the varying perceptions of different individuals at that Thanksgiving with you. Try talking to your sister, uncle, or cousin about Thanksgiving dinner. Their memories will be different from yours in important ways. What people wore or how they behaved may have had particular meanings to you that were significantly different from those of other family members.

Over time, you have undoubtedly found that your perception of these events changes. These changes may be attributed to many factors, one of which is learning. Learning has an impact on both the individual and culture. Additional information and experiences modify pre-existing personality, even though the underlying biology remains the same. As you mature, your interpretation and ultimately your memory of events at the family Thanksgiving change.

Memory is imperfect. We forget many events and reinterpret others on the basis of intervening occurrences (Brody, 2000). Mattingly (1998) suggests that rather than remembering experiences, we actually construct stories or narratives that represent those events. As new stories are incorporated into memory, they modify those previously constructed and the ways in which we interpret or construct narratives about the new experiences. Lynn and McConkey (1998) note that memories of childhood may change in certain details each time they are recalled in later life.

As an example of change in values over time based on personal experience, consider this story. One woman described how she had been raised to be prompt. In both her family and the surrounding culture, this was the norm. The woman adopted these values enthusiastically, even arriving early for appointments lest she be considered rude. Then the woman, a "Yankee," traveled to the southern United States as a young adult. She found herself extremely discomfited by the different perspective on time in that region. Life moved more slowly, promptness was not greatly valued, and she felt both out of place and annoyed by the seeming rudeness of those around her. Several years later, she went to Spain where she was surprised and dismayed to learn that she could not purchase a train ticket a day in advance. To her query, the ticket agent replied, "plenty of time tomorrow." This *mañana* time perspective caused her considerable anxiety; however, she also began to experience it as somewhat liberating, and she observed that she got on the train with no problem. By the time she later traveled to Guatemala, where lengthy meals and a general disregard for the clock were the norm, she found the pace a pleasant relief from her usual rigid schedule. She continues to be prompt in her business dealings, but she also recognizes the value of other perspectives and has, in her personal life, relaxed considerably, freeing herself and her friends from her previously rigid expectations. Her story or narrative about time changed as she incorporated new experiences into her earlier memories.

Differences in time perception among individuals and between cultures are not at all unusual. The Lees, raised in a Hmong agricultural community in Laos, could not tell time but recognized the crowing of a rooster. They rose early but could not have identified a set schedule for their days, responding instead to the demands of the agricultural calendar. In the United States they no doubt experienced conflict and difficulty as they adjusted to clock-based time and the different set of values associated with it. One of the most prominent conflicts between Native American and Western culture in the southwest United States also has to do with time; Native American children are often late to school, to the displeasure of their Western-raised teachers (England, 1986). Certainly, many Native American children learn to adapt to the expectations of the school, although it is a personal choice to do so. It is also a personal choice whether the new time perspective for school carries over to other aspects of daily life.

There is a complex interaction among personality characteristics, cultural constructs, and individual experience. Personality may cause an individual to be more or less inclined to value particular cultural attributes, but experience may alter those inclinations over time.

This kind of learning, both positive and negative, occurs constantly. All of us are incorporating new information and observations, reinterpreting previous ideas on the basis of that new information, and adjusting our actions and beliefs accordingly. Just as culture is emergent, so are our own identities emergent over time.

3-11. Can you identify an aspect of your identity that has changed over time? Have you experienced shifts in values or ways of spending time? **Q**

3-12. Think of yourself 5 years ago. In what ways would a description of you 5 years ago be different from how you would be described now?

Multicultural Strands Within Individuals in Heterogeneous Societies

As we have already noted, people exist in more than a single culture. Consider again the example of Thanksgiving. We all know that in the United States Thanksgiving is the fourth Thursday in November. Other cultures have thanksgiving celebrations at other times of year, and they take different forms. Jews celebrate their thanksgiving, *Sukkot*, in autumn and traditionally spend time in worship and reflection, both before and after their festive meal. The festive meal is unlikely to include turkey, although a roast chicken might appear on the table. The table itself will be located in a *sukkah*, a small outdoor hut constructed especially for the occasion from rough materials. Its ceiling is open to the sky, to commemorate the shacks in which Jewish ancestors lived while harvesting. For Orthodox Jews, the secular Thanksgiving might be just another day on the calendar; for less observant Jews, it may be another major holiday.

As established in Chapters 1 and 2, cultures do not include only those to which one belongs at birth. Nor are they all defined based on nationality and ethnicity. Professional cultures into which one enters as an adult may influence behavior. If one is a physician, professional culture may mean that Thanksgiving is punctuated by calls from the hospital. If one is a retailer, Thanksgiving may be the day of preparation for the biggest sales day of the year.

The interaction of cultures is a particularly fascinating phenomenon in a culturally diverse place like the United States. Recent immigrants bring with them the norms and beliefs of their country of origin but often find that those who have come before them have already incorporated some of the beliefs and behaviors of the United States into their practices. Alternatively, they may settle in particular geographic areas and alter the culture of that area significantly, as in the case of Cuban immigrants to South Florida. Over time, succeeding generations further modify cultural values, picking, choosing, and transforming what they absorb from the world around them. The extent to which an individual acquires new perspectives is partly a function of personality. Some immigrants readily acculturate in their new homes; others long for the "old country" and cling to its traditions.

Besides the phenomenon of acculturation, there is the impact of the increasing mix of multiple "minority" cultures in large urban areas. For example, Kosher Chinese restaurants are ubiquitous in New York, where large groups of Chinese and Jewish individuals have come in contact. Intermarriage among individuals from differing cultural, ethnic, or religious groups further complicates the picture.

Of course, culture has never been static. In every culture, change over time is inevitable. The Moorish invasion of Southern Spain in 711 AD forever changed the nature of the region, bringing new forms of art and architecture, new political and religious structures, new methods of calculation and agriculture, and new games and fashions. These influences, including some having to do with medicine and health, continued to intensify over 700 years of cultural contact. Because the majority of Spanish colonists to the western hemisphere in the early 16th century came from the region of Spain with the greatest Moorish influence, some of those influences were transported to the Americas, where they continue to be observable today. Similarly, the influx of Hmong refugees from Cambodia has altered the face of central California by altering food preferences, social service structures, and other aspects of daily life (Fadiman, 1997).

3-13. In your own community, what are the major ethnic, religious, or nationality groups represented? What groups come into the greatest amount of contact? What examples of acculturation have you noticed?

3-14. When you have time, drive or walk through some neighborhood where cultural groups different from your own mingle. Make notes about what you observe there that you do not see in your home neighborhood. Are there different types of stores, decorations, clothing, foods present, and languages used?

3-15. As part of developing your thinking as you read this book, you should begin to pay closer attention to national and world events that pertain to cultures and culture contact. Over the next few days, collect some news stories that discuss the effects of minority culture presence in the United States or international communities.

Dealing with Cultural Stereotypes

The interplay of personal and cultural factors, and of cultural factors from many cultures over time, leads to the conclusion that each individual has, in some important way, created his or her own culture. However, cultural stereotypes abound. **Stereotypes** are generalizations or categorizations about a particular group based on some common feature (e.g., appearance, ethnicity, gender, etc.). Stereotyping is a common phenomenon. Infants begin early to learn to categorize based on color, size, and shape, and our efforts to group phenomena continue throughout life. Categorization is a useful way to cope with the myriad stimuli that occur in our environment. Stereotyping groups of individuals is a way of extending the natural human tendency to categorize.

You probably can list dozens of such stereotypes yourself. Statements reflective of stereotypes often begin with phrases such as "Women are..." or "Italians all..." These stereotypes express the general observations we have made, read, or heard about that are believed to describe the group in question. Some stereotypes have some basis in reality as very broad, general group descriptors. There is, for example, increasing biological research to suggest that men and women are indeed different, and that, on average, women share particular traits with each other. The key is to recognize, as we have discussed, that although individuals may share traits, they are also unique. Individuals presenting themselves to you may or may not share some traits with your stereotypical image of the group from which they come; they certainly will not share all traits of that stereotype. In comparison with men in her culture, the average woman may be smaller, less physically strong, or more nurturing or collaborative. The particular woman with whom you are interacting, however, may be unusually strong, competitive, or individually aggressive.

Q 3-16. Take a moment to reflect on some of your own stereotypes. Recognizing that all people have such ideas, identify a particular category of individuals about whom you hold stereotypical views. How do you think you acquired those views? Do you know any people from that category? In what ways do those people conform to your stereotype? In what ways do they differ?

Most of us want to believe ourselves free of prejudice, and we believe that stereotyping is reflective of prejudice. We struggle to rid ourselves of those stereotypes, the struggle made more difficult by the fact that some stereotypes can reflect some level of observed patterning that is true of many

members of the particular group. However, acting on the basis of stereotypes is dangerous, as that truthful nugget may not apply at all to the particular group member with whom you are interacting; that person's individually patterned behavior must be considered instead.

Stereotypes are inevitable because they arise from fundamental features of human cognition: categorization and the identification of pattern. Stereotypes serve a useful purpose because they speed up cognitive processing, but their limitations must be acknowledged and understood. For example, clinical diagnoses are, in fact, stereotypes. Diagnostic categories have specific criteria. For example, rheumatoid arthritis is diagnosed when there are findings of morning stiffness, pain in three or more joints, joint pain in the hands, symmetrical joint pain, rheumatoid nodules, serum rheumatoid factor on laboratory testing, and radiographic changes (Arnett et al., 1988). However, all clinicians know that within the diagnostic group, individuals vary in terms of severity of the disorder and their reactions to it. Thus, the limitation of stereotypes is that they apply only in the most general way and never to everyone in a particular group or to any single individual in that group. A diagnosis of rheumatoid arthritis might tell you that the individual you are about to see has joint pain, but not about the severity of the pain or the disability. Further, the diagnosis will give you no information about the response of the individual to the rheumatoid arthritis. Both cultural and personal factors affect the degree to which pain is allowed to interfere with function for a given individual. There is no question that some cultures value stoicism and others value strong emotional expression. Research clearly demonstrates that individual and ethnic differences in experiences of pain and disability are significant (Bates & Edwards, 1992; Nayak et al., 2000).

Cultural and personal differences can be examined as related to particular experiences, such as reactions to pain. They can also be examined in the context of ethnic groupings. For example, knowing that someone is Hispanic provides only the most general of suppositions about the person, some, many, or all of which will or should be discarded upon meeting him or her. The Hispanic individual may come from Puerto Rico or Spain or Guatemala (in which case it may turn out that the supposed Hispanic person is actually Mayan). The individual may be a visitor to the mainland United States or a third-generation citizen residing in Indiana. The individual may speak Spanish or English as a first language and may or may not have a second language. The individual may be a professional, a laborer, or unemployed; male or female; old or young; an only child or youngest of six; shy or outgoing; bright or of average intelligence; and so on. Each added bit of information would alter your expectations about the person. Factoring in biological and personality factors would move reality even further away from your initial stereotype.

Sometimes, careful examination of a stereotype can provide valuable information about the dynamics of a situation. Consider the following example.

A friend recently described her son's high school graduation. She lived in a racially mixed community comprised mainly of upper middle class white and African-American families, with a smattering of individuals from Chinese and Japanese backgrounds, and a significant subset of Jewish families. She was a white, middle-aged woman from a Methodist background. She was very accomplished in both her work and family life, and was somewhat rigid and judgmental of others, expecting them to conform to her view of proper behavior. She described with outrage the "chaos" she experienced during the graduation ceremony, indicating that "some families do not know how to behave." The specific behavior that was upsetting to her was the loud cheering and applauding from many of the African-American families, which drowned out the speakers on stage and the names of students as they were read. The problem, as she described it, was that "those people are rude." Her stereotype gave her an explanation but no comfort in the situation.

It is tempting to respond to this person by saying, "They are not all rude. Some people of any background are rude," which is a true statement. However, more careful examination of cultural norms might reveal another explanation for the observed behavior. In some circles in the African-American community, participants in celebratory events signal their joy in an enthusiastic, overt, and noisy fashion. Worship by black congregations may be accompanied by shouted interaction between pastor and congregation, emotional singing, and "making a joyful noise." Parties can be exuberant affairs, and daily life is often characterized by spirited interaction. In fact, many individuals in this group would say that a celebration is not adequate unless it is accompanied by sufficient emotional expression.

Given this set of beliefs, the behavior of these families at the graduation could be recast as an expression of a particular cultural form of celebration. (It should be noted that in the South, many white middle-class families celebrate graduations in the same noisy fashion, so the patterns of ritual celebration are not necessarily distributed by "race.") That form of celebration is in direct conflict with another cultural expression of celebration, the Old American construction (Nayak et al., 2000), which is characterized by intense attention, respectful silence, and polite applause. It was the Old American form that the unhappy mother in this example preferred. There are no easy solutions to this particular dilemma—a case of cultural conflict during an important ritual. The two styles of ritual observance seem incompatible.

3-17. Can you think of some strategies that individuals might use to ameliorate the tensions inherent in this situation? What about strategies that the school or community might adopt? **Q**

It is inevitable that we develop stereotypes. Giving some thought to your own and recognizing the times they interfere with your ability to understand the individual in front of you can ameliorate some of the potential negative effects of such stereotyping.

3-18. Take a moment to think about one of your cultural attributes (e.g., an ethnic label or your professional affiliation). For that culture, list what you perceive to be the beliefs that others hold about that culture. In other words, identify the stereotypes for that culture. **Q**

3-19. Now consider the ways in which the stereotypes may be accurate (e.g., providing a general description of the culture). In what ways are they also inaccurate or overgeneralized?

3-20. Consider the following list of labels. Choose three labels and list in the notes some commonly held beliefs (stereotypes) about members of that group.

Appalachian	Mormons
White people	Ethiopians
French people	Texans
Finns	Jews
Yankees	Gay men
Black people	Costa Ricans

Q 3-21. Look over your list and think about the basis on which your stereotypes are formed. Personal observation? Popular media depictions? Parental comments? Reading? Have you known group members who did not conform to these stereotypical images?

3-22. Now think about why you chose the three groups you did. What role did familiarity play? What role did your own cultural sensitivities play?

Stereotyping can cause significant problems in clinical settings if it is not attended to carefully. Mattingly (1998) gives the example of Bob and Joe. A therapist had considerable success in treating Joe, a 26-year-old, working-class Irishman with two young children. When Bob arrived at the clinic, the therapist observed a 23-year-old, working-class Irishman with two young children, and was immediately reminded of Joe. On the basis of her superficial observations, the therapist proceeded to intervene with Bob in the manner that had been so effective with Joe. The intervention met with dismal failure, largely because the therapist's preconceived ideas based on superficial similarities made it difficult for her to appropriately recognize the differences between these two individuals.

Therapy and treatment, like all other human interaction, call for understanding where each individual came from, who he or she is, and what unique cultural and personal experiences have shaped his or her narratives. Although cultural stereotypes might give some hints about what to expect, effective therapists remain open to the potential for surprise. Recall that Sue (2000) underlines the importance of dynamic sizing skills, which enable you to determine when to generalize and when to individualize. He also recommends scientific-mindedness, the formation and testing of hypotheses that you can accept or discard based on carefully gathered evidence, as a means to acquire dynamic sizing skills.

Issues of Contact and Change

In the graduation example above, the contact between two cultures, influenced perhaps by personality, led to a misunderstanding with significant repercussions. The community in which the graduation took place is one that is trying to encourage diversity in its population. Careful measures have been taken to encourage mixing of cultural groups in their neighborhoods and everyday encounters. The community has received national attention for its efforts to accomplish this kind of interaction as a means to encourage understanding, reduce tension, and minimize discrimination. Obviously, contact does not always create harmony. The high school graduation exacerbated negative perceptions and generated considerable ill will. Perhaps the school might encourage greater sharing of information about cultural differences and personal expectations by organizing a meeting before the big event. Such a strategy could blunt some of the disappointment felt by individuals whose expectations are otherwise unmet, but it is unlikely that everyone can be satisfied.

The United States is a heterogeneous society. Multiple waves of immigration, both voluntary and involuntary, have brought people from all over the world to live here. In some cities, it is possible to walk from block to block as if one is moving from country to country, or even from one continent to another. Puerto Rican neighborhoods abut Vietnamese neighborhoods, just down the street from older Lithuanian neighborhoods. In communities that appear more homogeneous, it is likely that the white middle-class families come from an array of cultures of origin. In a single block, you might find Catholics, Protestants, Muslims, and Jews from families that emigrated from Ireland, Russia, Turkey, and England, some two generations ago, some eight generations ago, some last year. These families may find a great deal in common in their current situations; they will also have some important differences.

Intercultural contact can often occur relatively easily and have positive effects that everyone can enjoy. As a simple example, think of the rich musical variety in the United States, the result of influences from all over the world. African chants, Latin-American salsa, African-American gospel, and Appalachian folk music (originally of Celtic origin) have all influenced the wide array of musical styles found in this country, and music continues to change as international and intercultural exchange continues. Similarly, what we eat has undergone dramatic change, opening new dietary choices. As just one example, salsa has recently overtaken ketchup as the main condiment used in the United States. Think, too, of the influences of other cultures on health care in the United States. Meditation, massage, dietary balance, and other holistic concepts derive from centuries-old Far Eastern practices. Some of these practices have demonstrated value; for example, social support is of clear benefit in terms of quality of life and survival rates in cancer, a finding that might be predicted by traditional healers who place great value on balance and connection to others (Spiegel, Bloom, & Yalom, 1981).

Despite all the cultural influences on behavior, the importance of individual personality remains profound. The individual cultural expression, the culture emergent, that results from the interaction between culture and personality and between one person and another has profound impact on daily life and, as we shall see, on beliefs and values about health and health care.

✎ NOTES ✎

4

The Role of Culture in Health and Health Care

CHAPTER OBJECTIVES

By the end of the chapter, the reader will be able to:

1. Define health and sickness from a cultural perspective.
2. Discuss the relationship of culture to perceptions of the body.
3. Discuss the effect of culture on perceptions of the causation of sickness.
4. Define the concept of culture-bound syndrome.
5. Describe culture-bound syndromes found in Old American culture and in other cultures.
6. Discuss the ways in which individuals learn the roles associated with illness and disability.
7. Describe the role of health "self-care" in Old American and other cultures.
8. Describe characteristics of traditional healers and compare and contrast those with health care professionals in the United States.

THE STORY OF LIA LEE

The Lees had reasonably good experiences with Western medicine in their refugee camp in Thailand, where physicians saved three of their children. A fourth who had not been treated died. Therefore, when Lia had a seizure at 3 months of age, her parents carried her to the **community hospital** in Merced where she had been born.

Over the next few months, Lia had at least 20 more seizures, two of them so bad that her parents again carried her in their arms to the hospital. During the first two hospitalizations, no translator was available. One physician at the hospital observed that in such cases, because of the communication problem, he had to practice "veterinary medicine." Lung x-rays showed aspiration, misinterpreted as infection, that had occurred during a seizure; thus, antibiotics were given, along with seizure control medications. The Lees were concerned about the effects of the medications and unclear about the complex and constantly changing administration instructions. They were also worried about the multiple blood tests because the Hmong believe that the body has a finite amount of blood that can be depleted. Throughout these and subsequent hospitalizations, Foua stayed with Lia almost all the time. Foua carried Lia, caressed her, and spoke to her day and night during each hospital stay.

Among major illnesses identified by the Hmong are the following:

1. The presence of a *dab* or evil spirit master. The *dab* may cause illness by sucking blood or sitting on one's chest. A person can become ill by bumping into a *dab* living in a tree or stream, digging a well in a *dab*'s home, or catching sight of a *dab* in the forest.
2. Soul-loss, which occurs when a life-soul becomes separated from the body because of anger, grief, fear, or curiosity. Newborns are vulnerable to soul-loss from *dabs*.
3. *Nyuab Siab* (difficult liver), caused by loss of any item (e.g., home, status, family) that has a significant emotional value; its symptoms are worry, crying, confusion, delusions, and insomnia.
4. *Tu Siab* (broken liver). Caused by loss of or quarrel with a family member. The symptoms include grief, loneliness, guilt, and feelings of loss.

The Lees diagnosed Lia's problem as *qaug dab peg* (the spirit catches you and you fall down). In Hmong culture, *qaug dab peg* is considered both a problem and an honor. It made Lia special in their eyes, and she became the favorite of their beloved children. Meanwhile, the physicians continued to look for neurologic damage in Lia's brain, but were unable to identify a cause that would explain the seizures.

Lia's seizures continued with frequency, and changes in medication had no obvious effect. When she was 20 months, hospital personnel noted developmental delay. Members of the staff were worried that, as the seizures continued, these delays would become worse. The public health nurses who visited the child at home did not perceive the delays, perhaps because they saw her when she was well, not when she was sick.

During the third hospitalization, the Lees came with their cousin, who spoke some English. Medications were changed again to include Dilantin for the seizures and Ampicillin for the infection. Lia responded poorly to these and the many other medications that were prescribed during subsequent hospitalizations as her seizures continued, in part because medications were administered sporadically or in sub-therapeutic doses by her parents.

The Lees did not understand instructions given them in English (either spoken or written; they knew no English and were illiterate), nor did they approve of the side effects of the medications. In addition, they were confused by the frequent changes. Sometimes instead of or in addition to the prescribed medications, the Lees treated Lia with herbal remedies. They loved her greatly and spent a great deal of time holding and talking with her, caring for her scrupulously according to their traditions. Staff, who were monitoring blood levels of medications, felt that the Lees were noncompliant.

Summarized from Fadiman, A. (1997). *The spirit catches you and you fall down.* New York: Noonday Press.

INTRODUCTION

Perceptions of health and illness, as well as beliefs and values about health care, are all profoundly influenced by culture. Social roles and status positions, values, and rituals may all incorporate issues of health and illness. What is meant by health, how illness is defined, what constitutes disability, and assumptions about how illness is caused are all culturally defined. Likewise, views about how illness can be cured and who does the curing are influenced by cultural values and beliefs. Some of the most important rituals in cultures are those that protect against or treat illness. Some of the most important role and status delineations have to do with illness and curing. In addition to knowing about cultural aspects of daily life, health care providers must be aware of their clients' cultural values and beliefs as well as their personal feelings about health, sickness, and healing. Like the Lees, all individuals bring such beliefs to clinical encounters. Thus, to understand an individual's culture emergent, perceptions of illness and health must be explored.

Having articulated a model of culture and the relationship of culture and personality in Chapters 2 and 3, we now focus on the ways in which culture affects health and health care. An understanding of these relationships provides the basis for addressing the specifics of therapeutic care in **multicultural** settings in the remainder of this text.

UNDERSTANDING HEALTH AND SICKNESS

Sickness can be thought of as "an unwanted condition in one's person or self" (Hahn, 1995, p. 5). The concept of sickness can be applied cross-culturally because it is not tied to any specific cultural notion or artifact, such as the Western biomedical concept of disease. As Hahn notes, what counts is the perception and experience of the individual (e.g., one's subjective experience and values). Are you sick if you think you are, even if a physician can find no reason why you should feel sick? Hahn suggests that ill persons usually know when they are ill. One way to think about sickness is that it obstructs or threatens to obstruct everyday activities (Hahn, 1995). This approach is analogous to the notion of occupation employed by occupational therapists, who define occupation as all of the daily life tasks and activities in which an individual engages.

Throughout most health fields today, an increasingly accepted view holds that important health care outcomes emphasize the ability of an individual to accomplish important tasks and to experience satisfaction in life.

Thus, health can be defined as the absence of sickness or as the presence of desired abilities and self-defined good quality of life. Still, cultures may vary even around the issue of defining absence of sickness. In some cultures, when one is free of negative symptoms, one is not sick. In others, one may be sick if the body harbors certain organisms that can cause symptoms, even if one is disease-free at the moment. Such a difference in beliefs is one of many differences that has the potential to cause conflict in care situations, as individuals who hold the former belief may stop taking medication when symptoms disappear, whereas those who hold the latter belief may feel it important to continue medication until the organism is eradicated (DiversityRx, 1997b).

Likewise, definitions of good quality of life vary among cultures and among individuals. Many Native Americans tend to be somewhat stoical and consider pain and hardship to be part of life (Bell, 1995), whereas many Western cultures would find acceptance of such discomforts inconsistent with good quality of life.

4-1.   How do you define "quality of life"? What types of health conditions do you think would interfere so greatly in your life that you would not enjoy good quality of life? What activities do you consider essential to your well-being?

4-2.   How does your profession define health and sickness? In your discipline, who decides whether a person is sick: the person, the person's family, the person's physician? Are there cases where the patient does not notice any symptoms but can still be considered sick?

Perceptions of the Body and the Environment

One of the bases of beliefs about health is one's perception of the body. How you perceive your body is grounded through enculturation and influenced by individual experiences and personality. Individual cultures have varying perceptions of the nature of the body, its frailties and strengths, as well as the ways in which it is susceptible to sickness. In addition, each culture has particular notions about

Figure 4-1. Antigua sin barreras (Antigua without barriers). A modern concept is superimposed on a centuries-old city.

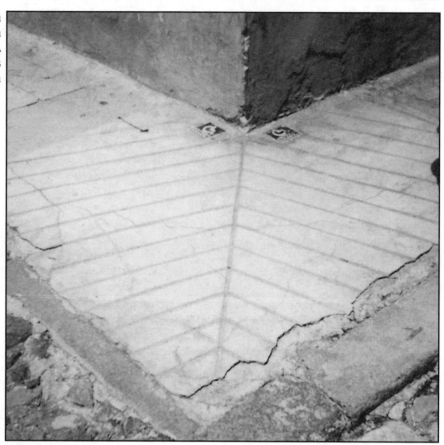

how the body changes and how it can be fixed or repaired when illness or injury occurs.

The relationship of the body to the environment is also seen through a cultural screen. Almost every culture has some beliefs about elements in the environment (e.g., spirits, toxic substances, evil humors, germs) that contribute to illness and injury. Culturally defined ideas about the body in the environment address a multitude of questions: Is the body in balance with nature? Is nature the source of healing? Is the environment hostile to the body?

Q

4-3. Review your own beliefs about the body and good health. What elements in the environment do you consider bad for your health? Which elements are good, contributing to your good health? What contributes most to the body's susceptibility to illness or injury? What role does mental attitude play?

4-4. Thinking of various cultural influences that affect you, can you identify some beliefs or perceptions specifically related to health? Can you identify some competing perceptions about the body? How do you resolve these competing perceptions?

4-5. Consider Figure 4-1. How might this particular environment affect the beliefs about, and realities of, physical disability?

Perceptions of the Causation of Sickness

Culture is the primary factor determining one's understanding of the causation of sickness. Western health care has a primarily **biomedical** or mechanical view of illness. This view holds that structural and biological agents cause illness. Germs and viruses cause illnesses such as those labeled common cold, tuberculosis, and acquired immunodeficiency syndrome (AIDS). Emotional difficulties are caused by imbalance in neurotransmission. Paralysis is caused by severed or damaged nerves. Treatment, therefore, is with drugs to kill the germs or alter the neurotransmitters, and with surgery to reconnect nerves or to implant sensors providing stimuli to the damaged nerve. Although widely accepted in the United States and Europe, these are far from the only views on the causes of illness. Even among practitioners working primarily in settings supportive of the Western model, there are varying views on the causation of illness.

Q   4-6. Think for a moment about your own profession. How does it define or explain sickness and disability?

Because health is so central to life, all cultures have constructed some beliefs about how one should behave to avoid illness and how to treat illness when it occurs. For example, a disability may be construed as a physical impairment that can and should be treated with surgery, or as a functional problem that can be addressed using environmental modifications, or even as a psychological problem best remediated by recasting of the disability. These beliefs come from many sources, and each of us carries messages from several of these sources.

Q   4-7. Think, for example, about your own beliefs about the common cold. What causes colds, in your opinion? How can you best avoid colds? What is the best treatment for colds?

You probably know that colds are caused by a virus and you may even know that there are many strains of cold-causing rhinovirus. Most medical personnel believe that such viruses are transmitted primarily through hand-to-hand contact and can be avoided by frequent hand-washing. Perhaps you also think you should avoid drafts in the winter. Have you ever been advised not to go outside in winter with your hair wet? Although scientifically discredited, these are widely held beliefs among many cultural groups; and for many people in the United States, including well-educated ones, they compete with the germ model as motivators of everyday behavior and as explanations for the onset of a cold.

One current example of the potential for conflict in health beliefs about causation is reflected in reports from the 2000 International Conference on AIDS. Western medicine is firmly agreed that the cause of AIDS is human immunodeficiency virus (HIV); however, some groups are convinced that the virus is unrelated to the disease and that its cause lies elsewhere ("A Turning Point for AIDS?", 2000). The dispute is frustrating to Western medical practitioners who want to implement aggressive prevention practices that are perceived by the other groups as useless and inappropriate.

Another example comes from the realm of mental health. The causes of depression are complex. Some health professions emphasize a biological cause agent: faulty neurotransmitter chemistry in the brain. Others emphasize other causes, whether based on environment (e.g., childhood experiences, situational stress), personality (e.g., perfectionistic, obsessive), or cognition (e.g., distorted thinking, habitual negative response patterns). For depressed patients, these conflicts among providers may affect care, and the power of the biomedical brain chemistry model is so strong that reimbursement decisions may favor drugs over talk as the preferred therapeutic strategy.

Sometimes fundamental differences in perception of causation can have profound impact on the course of treatment. The case of Lia Lee demonstrates the tragic consequences of cultural misunderstanding between a family of Hmong immigrants to the United States and the physicians and nurses who try to treat their daughter's severe epilepsy, characterized by frequent, lengthy grand mal seizures that had delayed her language acquisition and motor development. The parents assigned one kind of cause and the health professionals another. Perception of cause led to identification of relevant treatments, again strikingly different. Lack of shared information, misunderstanding of the perspective of the other participants, and disappointed expectations on all sides each contributed to problematic interactions and less successful outcomes.

4-8. Reread the segment of the Lees' story that opens this chapter. Identify as many points of conflict as you can. Which do you think may lead to major problems as the story unfolds?   **Q**

Cultural conflicts about health beliefs can lead to a loss of faith in the clinician. If a person believes that a health problem is caused by cold drafts or excessive heat build-up in the body, he or she may feel that the therapist who applies a drug treatment is using inappropriate practices. The provider who observes the care recipient engaging in an incomprehensible (to the provider's eyes) ceremony to foil the evil eye will almost certainly denigrate the superstitious nature of that procedure.

Cultural Constructions of Sickness

Culture defines not only what causes sickness, but also how sickness is demonstrated. For example, as noted in Chapter 3, objective pain appears to be similar among individuals regardless of culture (Nayak et al., 2000), but behavioral expression of pain differs significantly. Some cultures consider overt expression not only acceptable but expected; others feel that stoicism is preferable. Nayak et al. found that college students from India were much less likely to express pain openly than were

American college students. Among cultural groups in the United States, the group we call Old Americans (following the researchers' example) were least expressive, whereas individuals from recently arrived Hispanic families were most expressive; other cultures formed a well-distributed continuum between these two groups (Bates & Edwards, 1992). The interpretation of the pain experience differs as well. In Filipino culture, pain is perceived not only as part of life, but also as an opportunity to atone for past sins (Mattson & Lew, 1991). There is also evidence that individual experience and expression of pain is mediated by personality factors (APA, 1994), so that within cultural groups such as Old Americans or Hispanics a good bit of individual variability will exist.

Q 4-9. As in earlier chapters, we have used the label Old American to identify the mainstream cultural group in the United States. We asked you earlier to reflect on your image of that group and to think about what else the group might be called. Take a moment now to reflect on the health beliefs of that group. Use the Notes section to record a few of them.

4-10. How do you know that those are the dominant beliefs? (Consider the messages of media such as television commercials for drugs or movies with health issues as topics.) Do those beliefs conform to your own? In what ways are they similar? In what ways do they diverge?

One learns to express one's illness through observation and direct instruction. You have surely seen mothers at the playground reacting differently to children's scraped knees. One brushes it off and sends the child back to play; another coos and cuddles the child and expresses worry. Such strategies provide strong lessons to the child about how pain is to be addressed; undoubtedly, their parents learned such lessons from their parents as well.

4-11. Recall your own early childhood experiences of pain. In your family, how did adults tend to react to injury or illness? Can you identify patterns in your own behavior as an adult that may be related to those early models (whether you adopted or rejected them)? As you grew older did you develop different values about pain based on other experiences—e.g., by playing organized sports? **Q**

LEARNING TO BE A LEPER

We began with a bacillus, mildly communicable, treatable, not life-threatening, nor even deforming if treated early. Now we see that the bacillus itself is only a minor actor in the drama of leprosy. Instead, surrounding the disease in many societies is a set of social beliefs and expectations that profoundly affect the patient's experience and the doctor's work.

First we showed that the stigma of leprosy is not universal. In many societies, even where leprosy is common, leprosy is believed to be just another of the debilitating illnesses that many families must tolerate. Patients remain at home and marriages continue. In other societies, lepers are quickly divorced, pushed out of their homes, to end up as beggars. This cross-cultural variation in the stigma of leprosy led us to conclude that the source of a particular response is in the social and cultural matrix in which the disease exists.

In many societies beliefs about leprosy developed and stabilized long before written records were kept. In 19th-century Hawaii, however, we saw the economic and social threat of the Chinese immigrants become transformed into the social threat of the disease they were believed to carry. In Africa, we pointed to the beginning of what could be a new, and stigmatized, notion of leprosy inadvertently introduced by public health educators. Thus, the moral definition of leprosy may arise from particular historical/social/medical circumstances different in each society.

Second, we showed that the ideology surrounding leprosy provides a map for the leper. Moral definitions tell the leper how to 'have' the illness. We contrasted Ethiopian and American experiences, profoundly different, but each exemplifying the effect of society's expectations on the leper's career.

From Wexler, N. E. (1981). Learning to be a leper. In E. G. Mishler et al. (Eds.), *Social contexts of health, illness and patient care* (p. 156). Cambridge, England: Cambridge University Press. Reprinted with permission.

Q 4-12. If you experienced a serious illness or disability as a child—or know well someone who did—what further lessons were learned about sickness, disability, and health care?

Learning also occurs as individual situations change. Newly disabled individuals experience feelings of alienation as they must reinvent themselves within a disability culture (Luborsky, 1994). Murphy (1987) describes the increasing physical limitations that resulted from a slow-growing spinal tumor. His own view was that he was not disabled, as through trial and error (but unfortunately not through the services of therapists) he continued to accomplish all the daily activities that were important to him. The health care world, however, and many others around him, identified him as disabled and, in his view, discounted his abilities. In the United States there is a tendency to view disability in a way that devalues continuing competencies, autonomy, and achievements (Luborsky, 1994). Sometimes such perceptions persist even when the disease or disability itself may have undergone a profound shift as a result of new treatments. Notice on the previous page how Wexler (1981) describes the situation of individuals with Hansen's disease (leprosy) and the process of "learning to be a leper". This process is characterized by the individual's tendency to isolate him- or herself from society, even though new treatments for leprosy and understanding of its causes and spread make it clear that this is unnecessary.

Conflicting perceptions about the nature of disability, such as those Wexler describes, can have profound effects on the effectiveness of intervention.

Q 4-13. Given that Chinese immigrants seem to have been perceived as a threat by the population of Hawaii, how do you think leprosy was perceived there? Do you think that individuals with leprosy were more likely to remain in their homes or to be ostracized under those circumstances?

4-14. What other diseases can you think of that might carry different connotations in different cultures? What about injuries or birth defects? Make a few notes about your ideas.

4-15. Consider what you know and have observed about people with chronic health conditions. Can you think of examples that support the notion of "learning how to be" ill or disabled?

4-16. As you have aged or watched older people in your family do so, you have no doubt observed changes in health status, physical ability, or functional capacity. How have these changes affected the sense of personal identity or perceived quality of life? Do you think it is accurate to say that people "learn to be old"?

Culture-Bound Syndromes

The anthropological literature contains many examples of "diseases" that seem to be specific to a single culture or a group of related cultures. *Amok* among the Malay, *koro* among some Chinese, and *susto* in some Spanish-speaking cultures are examples of sicknesses that are widely known as **culture-bound syndromes** (see definitions in box below).

SOME CULTURE-BOUND SYNDROMES

Amok: A mental/emotional affliction known in the Philippines that causes one to become a killer.

Koro: An affliction described in China and Southeast Asia in which the genitalia are perceived to be shrinking and withdrawing into the body; death is the eventual outcome.

Susto: An ailment widely associated with Spanish-speaking groups in Europe as well as North and South America in which the soul is believed to leave the body as a result of a frightening event.

Adapted from American Psychiatric Association. (1994). *Diagnostic and statistical manual of mental disorders* (4th ed.). Washington, DC: Author.

DIAGNOSTIC CRITERIA FOR PREMENSTRUAL DISPHORIC DISORDER

A. In most menstrual cycles during the past year, five (or more) of the following symptoms were present for most of the time during the last week of the luteal phase, began to remit within a few days after the onset of the follicular phase, and were absent in the week post-menses, with at least one of the symptoms being either (1), (2), (3), or (4):

1. Markedly depressed mood, feelings of hopelessness, or self-deprecating thoughts
2. Marked anxiety, tension, feelings of being "keyed up," or "on edge"
3. Marked affective lability (e.g., feeling suddenly sad or tearful or increased sensitivity to rejection)
4. Persistent and marked anger or irritability or increased interpersonal conflicts
5. Decreased interest in usual activities (e.g., work, school, friends, hobbies)
6. Subjective sense of difficulty in concentrating
7. Lethargy, easy fatigability, or marked lack of energy
8. Marked change in appetite, overeating, or specific food cravings
9. Hypersomnia or insomnia
10. A subjective sense of being overwhelmed or out of control
11. Other physical symptoms such as breast tenderness or swelling, headaches, joint or muscle pain, a sensation of "bloating," weight gain

B. The disturbance markedly interferes with work or school or with usual social activities or relationships with others (e.g., avoidance of social activities, decreased productivity and efficiency at work or school).

C. The disturbance is not merely an exacerbation of the symptoms of another disorder, such as major depressive disorder, panic disorder, dysthymic disorder, or a personality disorder (although it may be superimposed on any of these disorders).

D. Criteria A, B, and C must be confirmed by prospective daily ratings during at least two consecutive symptomatic cycles (the diagnosis may be made provisionally prior to this confirmation).

From American Psychiatric Association. (1994). *Diagnostic and statistical manual of mental disorders* (4th ed., p. 717). Washington, DC: Author. Reprinted with permission.

Q

4-17. Do you think *amok* might be useful in explaining episodes of fatal school violence in the United States?

4-18. How does the Western biomedical model consider the possible impacts of extremely frightening events? Do you think *susto* and post-traumatic stress disorder (PTSD) might have anything in common?

Western cultures also have syndromes that might be considered culture-bound, although Western medical science may not treat them as culturally defined. Practitioners can provide elaborate descriptions of such disorders. For example, it can be argued that premenstrual syndrome (PMS) is a culture-bound syndrome that may not exist outside the Western world. (See diagnostic criteria in box above.)

Premenstrual disphoric disorder (commonly termed PMS) is rarely encountered in other cultures, although it is believed to be widespread among Euro-American women. This distribution alone might lead someone to offer it as an example of a culture-bound syndrome.

4-19. What evidence would you want in order to decide whether PMS is culture-bound?

Q

4-20. If a woman has many of the symptoms listed under criterion A but does not believe they interfere with her daily life (criterion B), might she still subjectively consider herself sick? Might others? How might your responses relate to the notion that illness is both culturally and personally constructed?

Q 4-21. How important is it, do you think, to determine the culture-boundedness of a sickness?

Within a given culture, experiences of a culture-bound syndrome are psychologically and physically real and the causes and cures are widely agreed upon; outside the culture, the affliction, even as a set of symptoms, may be unknown. Thus such afflictions are difficult for outsiders to understand or explain. Sometimes those outside the culture where the affliction is known resort to their own explanatory systems in an attempt to understand it and to attribute causation. Consider the following example.

In the 19th century, many cultures residing close to the North American arctic circle (e.g., Inuit and Aleut groups) suffered from an affliction described in the ethnographic literature as *pribloqtoq*. In its common form, an individual in a kayak would perceive that the boat was about to capsize and the only recourse was to remain perfectly still. Unless the kayak floated toward shore or unless another individual saw that the afflicted person was in trouble, the sufferer might be lost as he or she floated out to sea. If the afflicted one was rescued, he or she was likely to suffer future attacks until one proved fatal. In the Western psychological literature, this affliction is sometimes called *kayakangst*.

Some have attempted to explain *pribloqtoq* as a culturally specific expression of mental disease. The sufferers are mentally ill and the expression of their illness is culturally constructed. Many phobias that are common in Western culture are likewise culture bound; for example, school phobia occurs only where school is a typical and expected activity. Others have looked toward physiological or environmental conditions, such as calcium deficiency, to explain the *pribloqtoq*.

It is typical to assume that culture-bound syndromes have a high degree of psychological or religious overtone (Neff, 1997). As in the case of *kayakangst*, disorders commonly identified in Hispanic cultures including *aire*, *empacho*, *calda de la mollera*, *ojo*, and *susto* are all thought by Western practitioners to be psychosocial in origin. That is, they are believed to have no biological cause, such as bacteria.

Q 4-22. Consider the case of Lia Lee and the Hmong diagnosis of *qaug dab peg*. What factors might lead you to consider this condition to be a culture-bound syndrome, on the basis of what you know so far? (Keep in mind that you would need to know a great deal more to confirm this label.)

If we reverse the perspective and examine syndromes identified in Old American culture, we say that large numbers of these individuals suffer from illnesses that are largely unknown in the rest of the world.

ADOLESCENCE AS A CULTURE-BOUND SYNDROME

Adolescent "storm and stress" (*sturm und drang*) appears to be primarily a Western construct. It is described in much of the research literature as having three key elements:

- Conflict with parents
- Mood disturbance
- Risk behavior

Current evidence suggests that biological change contributes to these behaviors. Hormonal changes can certainly contribute to mood disruption. However, there is also evidence that delayed phase preference may be a factor. This phenomenon has to do with biorhythms, which, in adolescents, support rising late in the morning and staying up late at night. In Western societies, where an early start to the school day is common, lack of sleep may result in a sleep-deprived state.

In less developed cultures, storm and stress may be lower because of cultural rather than biological differences. Globalization may increase this adolescent reaction in those other cultures.

Adapted from Arnett, J. J. (1999). Adolescent storm and stress, reconsidered. *American Psychologist*, 54, 317-326.

Anorexia nervosa (Banks, 1992) and obesity fit the criteria of culture-bound syndromes. *Anorexia nervosa* is not only most common in Western cultures, but in particular subgroups within those cultures, notably gymnasts, ballet dancers, and wrestlers. Some have argued that adolescence as we experience it in the United States is a culture-bound syndrome (Hill & Fortenberry, 1992), as it does not appear in cultures in which children move immediately to marriage and work in their early teenage years. Consider this idea further by reviewing the box on page 67.

Hahn (1995) disputes the concept of culture-bound syndrome altogether, finding it not only unhelpful but also misleading. Hahn feels that culture-bound syndromes are always mental conditions, and that the exclusionist understanding of culture-bound syndromes implicit in the term distorts the role of culture and of physiology in human affairs. Whatever view you adopt toward the existence of such culture-bound syndromes, the underlying issue is of vital importance. Individuals from different cultures perceive and experience illness within the context of their cultural backgrounds. These experiences are not uniform, and attempts to discount them will lead to significant dilemmas in their treatment.

THE RELATIONSHIP OF CULTURE AND HEALTH CARE

Self-Care and Health Practices Cross-Culturally

Culture, individual experience, and personality all may have an impact on perceptions and behaviors related to self-care and health practices. Such practices include personal hygiene, diet, and exercise, as well as safety practices and illness-avoidance practices. The chosen behaviors may be in direct conflict with Western medical perceptions. For example, among Amish women, obesity (as defined by Western medicine) is prevalent (Purnell & Paulanka, 1998). In this culture, food is an important aspect of celebration, and, because of the intense agricultural work done by the men, it is also associated with perceptions about maintaining one's strength. Women, however, do less strenuous physical work, and they experience frequent pregnancies. The Amish do not necessarily perceive the resultant high body weight of the women as a health problem; in fact it may be viewed positively,

as a means to "keep up one's strength." This kind of belief would reduce the value of commonly recommended weight-reduction strategies in Western medicine, such as education about "proper" body weight and ideal nutrition.

In fact, food is an area in which self-care beliefs are profoundly influenced by culture. Dietary self-care practices influence the amounts and kinds of food eaten, times in the life cycle when special diets are needed (e.g., infancy, pregnancy, old age), balance among food groups, and foods to avoid. In Western societies, people focus on the latest scientific findings, believing that through science, "right" answers about food can be found. This emphasis often may leave people puzzled about observations in conflict with these scientific findings. For example, the French are perceived as eating a diet too high in fat, and they are known to consume a considerable amount of alcohol, and yet the French have a relatively low rate of heart disease. Scientific research had claimed that alcohol was bad for health, as was excessive fat. Many people in the United States breathed a sigh of relief when science "explained" the contradiction by determining that wine in moderate quantities protects against heart disease.

4-23. Can you think of other relationships between culture and food, as related to health? Think about the fundamental definition of what is edible and what is not. From the following list, mark with a "+" those items you accept as food for humans, even if you yourself do not eat them. Then mark with an "x" those items you think people in some cultures eat but that you could never eat. Mark with "0" those items you think no one anywhere would ever eat.

____ Rat meat	____ Acorns
____ Liver	____ Whale blubber
____ Octopus	____ Dog meat
____ Yucca plant flowers	____ Nettles
____ Grubs	____ Thistle
____ Grasshoppers	____ Ham

4-24. All these items are or have been considered food someplace in the world. Do the items you could not eat form any sort of grouping or belong to any specific categories? Do those categories have any cultural significance?

4-25. Do the items you thought would never be considered food fall into any definable group?

How does that grouping reflect your own cultural categories?

In terms of personal hygiene, culture influences when one bathes, what kind of water is used, special types of baths (e.g., sweat baths), type and weight of clothing, special care of specific body parts (e.g., eyes or teeth), and habits around elimination of body wastes.

Q 4-26. List some of the rules you observe about caring for your teeth. How often do you brush? How often do you change toothbrushes? What kind of toothbrush do you use? Do you floss? Do you crunch unpopped popcorn kernels? How often do you see a dentist?

4-27. Return to the Miner article in Chapter 1 on the Nacirema and reread the description of the mouth-rite and the holy-mouth-men. How culture-bound do you think your dental care rules are?

Self-care and prevention may also emphasize the emotional and spiritual realms. In many cultures, there are specific guidelines about avoidance of negative emotions such as jealousy that may cause emotional unbalance or physical illness. In others, amulets are worn to protect against the evil eye. The Lees used hats to protect Lia from *dabs* (evil spirits). Similarly, Mayan families believe it is important to protect infants with close-fitting red hats, not to let pregnant women or anyone outside the immediate family look at the infant for several days after birth, and to burn incense to keep evil spirits away.

For a good example of the interaction of cultural beliefs about causality, prevention, and treatment of illness, consider the widely used **hot-cold system**, one of the most prevalent folk medical systems found in many Latino, African, and a number of Caribbean cultures, as well as in the southern United States. Review the description of this system in the box that begins below.

THE HOT-COLD SYSTEM OF HEALTH MAINTENANCE

The basic structure of hot-cold beliefs suggests that certain substances in the environment and the individual can be classified as hot or cold. It seems likely that belief in this model is as old as Hippocratic theory in Greece—from around 460 BCE (Foster & Anderson, 1978). Hippocrates elaborated on earlier work by the Greek physician Galen (c 130-200), which claimed that the body had four humors—hot, cold, wet, and dry—that operated in balance with each other. Good health was characterized by equilibrium; lack of balance resulted in illness. As travel among cultures occurred, these beliefs were dispersed, as well. Foster and Anderson (1978) traced them from Greece to Egypt, then to the Byzantine Empire. From there, the beliefs were carried to Persia, to Pakistan and Malaysia, to Africa, and to Spain by the Moors. From Africa, the beliefs moved across the ocean to the Caribbean, and from Spain to Central and South America. Along the way, they were transmuted based on the memories of travelers, local beliefs, time, and experience. At least some of the four elements posited by Hippocrates appear in health care beliefs in many cultures around the world. However, the details of those beliefs vary, even in regions we might consider closely related.

In most areas where these beliefs are found, the elements wet and dry have disappeared or have been incorporated into other categories, leaving the hot–cold balance as the focus of concern. Most typically, the hot–cold system is a categorization of objects and processes. Certain types of foods may be considered cold, others hot. The categorization does not refer to the actual temperature of the food but to a variety of other factors. For example, among peoples of the Mexican Yucatan peninsula, tubers are considered cold foods because they feel cold and are grown in the cold ground (McCullough, 1973). In Tecospa, in the Valley of Mexico, ice is considered hot because it burns the skin; boiling water is considered cold because the initial sensation is of cold (Masden, 1955).

continued

As a health maintenance strategy, this system is predicated on the need to maintain the appropriate balance between hot and cold elements or substances. Illness resulting from a lack of balance must be treated with substances of the appropriate category. However, just as the classification of elements as hot or cold varies from location to location, so do treatment recommendations. In Tecospa, excessive heat is to be treated by introducing cold (Masden, 1955). For example, a sprain (cold) should be treated by application of raw weasel meat (hot). A black widow spider bite (cold) should be treated with black coffee (hot). In this location, two additional temperatures, "brisk" and "temperate," have been added to the system, and sometimes treatment requires application of an element of one of these temperatures. The system also accommodates and categorizes imported items. Thus, headache (hot) may be treated with aspirin (temperate).

In the Yucatan, the system recommends avoiding application of opposite temperature. After working in the fields (hot), individuals should avoid drinking water (cold) unless salt (hot) is added. It is tempting to read this description and assume that the hot-cold system has evolved to reflect current Western medical wisdom in that salt depletion is a problem in dehydration so adding salt to water ameliorates this problem. Such influences have undoubtedly taken place, although it is often difficult to establish the precise mechanisms.

Folk remedies, as with any remedy, cannot necessarily be assumed to be 100% effective. There are times that the hot–cold classification leads to damage. In Haiti, for example, maternal malnutrition during lactation leads to significant infant mortality. Wiese (1976) notes that of 37 foods available to rural Haitians, 27 (including river fish, mango, avocado, grapefruit, lime juice, and sweet potato) are forbidden for lactating women. Maternal malnutrition, then, is probably not only based on the impoverished economic conditions, but also on the use of hot–cold classifications to determine what foods are safe to eat during lactation. The resulting diet is severely deficient in important nutrients.

During a recent visit to Guatemala, one of us was asked to assist a girl who had developed a rash. When a tube of cortisone cream was produced, there was much discussion about whether this cure was hot or cold and whether the disorder was hot or cold. When the villagers were informed that it would be important to keep the girl out of the sun while using the cream, there were many knowing nods about too much heat, an insight that clarified the nature of the cure as "hot."

Q 4-28. Think back to the earlier exercise about the causes of colds. Some people, perhaps people you know, think that upper respiratory infections can be caused by sitting in a draft. What relationship do you think this could have to the hot–cold belief system? How do you think such a belief could have entered Old American culture?

Ideas of balance are common in many cultures. In Ayurvedic medicine practiced in India and in Chinese medicine, balance is a vital component of health. Whether defined as yin-yang or hot-cold, the notion that there is a particular natural state in which complementary forces support good health is widespread. Such systems exhibit an internal flexibility that allows them to adjust to changing contexts and thus persist over centuries and across wide distances. Hot-cold belief systems are quite flexible and continue to incorporate new information, such as diagnoses, and new treatment options, such as imported medicines. Note that the generalized inventory shown in the box on the next page includes both Western disease names and modern medicines.

Health Care Specialists Cross-Culturally

Just as each culture has its explanations of illness and healing, each also has health care specialists who provide treatment when self-care fails. These specialists have specific attributes and defined levels of status within the culture. In Western medicine, practitioners include physicians; psychologists; physical, occupational, and speech therapists; nurses; and social workers. Each has a particular role, and there is a clear hierarchy of status, with physicians at the top.

Western influence has spread to many cultures, but alternative traditions remain. *Curanderos*, shamans, and other kinds of healers are prominent

SOME HOT AND COLD CONDITIONS AND TREATMENTS IN MEXICAN-AMERICAN CULTURE

Hot Conditions	Cold Conditions
Fever	Cancer
Infections	Pneumonia
Diarrhea	Malaria
Kidney problems	Joint pain
Hot Foods	**Cold Foods**
Chocolate	Fresh vegetables
Cheese	Tropical fruits
Eggs	Dairy products
Peas	Honey
Hot Medicines and Herbs	**Cold Medicines and Herbs**
Penicillin	Orange flower water
Tobacco	Linden
Ginger root	Milk of magnesia
Garlic	

Adapted from Giger, J. N., & Davidhizar, R. E. (1991). *Transcultural nursing: Assessment and intervention.* St. Louis: Mosby.

in Hispanic, African, and Asian cultures, among others. Their healing traditions have continued to prosper among immigrant communities in the United States. In the Southwest and in cities with large Hispanic populations, it is possible to find *curanderos* and other specialists in active practice. *Curanderos* are usually at the top of the hierarchy, with *yerberos* (herbalists), *sobadores* (massage specialists), and *parteras* (midwives) next, and *señoras* or *abuelas* (older wise women) following (Neff, 1997) (Figures 4-2 and 4-3).

Individuals must make choices among care providers, including both traditional and Western ones. Such choices are typically based on a number of factors, including the individual's perception of what is wrong. If the individual suspects having a condition or syndrome most amenable to traditional interventions, he or she is likely to seek out a traditional healer. In the United States, this choice is not incompatible with use of a Western provider for other conditions (Figure 4-4).

Such choices are made by most individuals, even those who do not necessarily subscribe to beliefs about traditional healing. For example, in Western tradition, low back pain may be treated by an orthopedic surgeon, a physical therapist, or a chiropractor, among others. Individual beliefs will dic-

tate which of these healers is sought first, and the outcomes of that intervention may affect future choices. Increasingly, other traditional healers are being added to the list of possible therapists for back pain. Acupuncturists, masseurs, and hypnotherapists may all be sought to provide relief. Individuals from non-Western cultures may find themselves puzzled by this wide array of unfamiliar kinds of practitioners just as Westerners confronted by herbalists, curers, and diviners might also be confused.

4-29. Reflect on your own opinions about traditional or alternative health care specialists. Have you ever consulted an alternative provider? Do you know what kinds of traditional specialists practice in your community? How does your profession view alternative practitioners and practice?

Q

Many traditional healers, Hispanic *curanderos* for example, believe in and support an array of Western interventions. They may well refer cases to a physician or encourage a patient to follow-through on recommendations made by a physician. A Mayan bonesetter—a specialist who treats fractures and dislocations—described how he determined whether to treat individuals seeking his care.

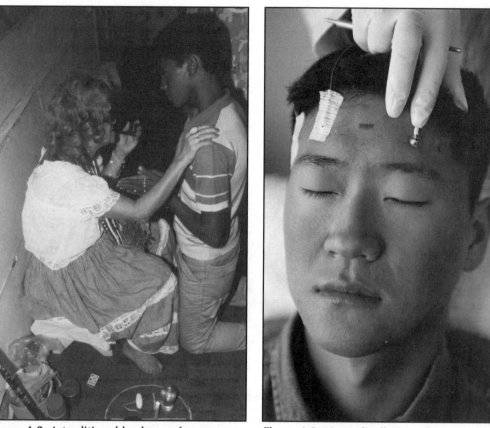

Figure 4-2. A traditional healer performs a curing ceremony in Brazil. Photo courtesy of Douglas Bryant.

Figure 4-3. Biomedically-based healing involves different technologies.

He indicated that a careful assessment of the problem came first. If a bone was clearly broken and the fracture was compound (breaking the skin), he always referred the individual to a Western physician. If the problem was clearly a soft-tissue injury, he was likely to treat the problem without referral. Other problems fell on a continuum between these two points. An additional factor in his referral practices was the faith that the individual expressed in his methods. As he put it, "If they don't believe I can help, I won't be able to."

Just as orthopedic surgeons and physical therapists have differing approaches to treatment of low back pain, traditional curers have differing approaches to health problems. To treat an upper respiratory infection, an herbalist might suggest the following treatment regimen: restrict dairy products; take vitamins C and B and zinc; and ingest chamomile, elderflower, catmint, and echinacea. A *curandero* might recommend teas: sage, gordolobo, eucalyptus, and oregano (Neff, 1997). The suggested substances appear to have some common attributes, and there is evidence that they can be helpful

in symptomatic treatment of upper respiratory infection. It is useful to recall that Western healers are also restricted to providing symptomatic relief, as there currently is no cure for viral upper respiratory infection.

The array of healers in Western culture can be confusing to those from other cultures (Purnell & Paulanka, 1998). Such professions as physical therapy, occupational therapy, social work, and speech therapy may not exist in some countries and cultures (Queensland Government, 1998). The Lees, the Hmong family described throughout this book, solved the dilemma by identifying all their daughter's care providers as "Lia's doctors."

CULTURAL DOMAINS IN CLINICAL ENCOUNTERS

In addition to beliefs about causes of illness, there are many alternative beliefs about interventions. In the United States, there is increasing support for the use of an array of herbal and folk reme-

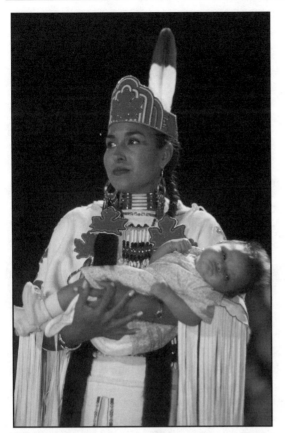

Figure 4-4. Kiowa ceremonies may incorporate concepts of health or healing.

dies. Echinacea, St. John's wort, ginkgo, and other herbs are now sold in grocery and drug stores, having become mainstream "cures." In spite of efforts by the U.S. Food and Drug Administration to call their effectiveness into doubt, so-called natural remedies are currently growing in popularity (i.e., value) among consumers. At the same time, increased skepticism is being expressed about Western medical models for cure.

This change in perception extends to other forms of medical intervention as well. For example, many individuals are attempting to control pain through acupuncture or meditation, rather than through surgery or drugs. This observation does not mean that Western medicine has been discarded. Rather, it means that in terms of both causation and remediation, a single individual may hold divergent, sometimes even conflicting, views. These views come from the multiple experiences that influence the individual. These differences are not a matter of who is right and who is wrong. This fact is of considerable importance to you as a health care provider.

Among the beliefs inherent in Western health care is the infallibility of science. Thus, interventions not "proved" scientifically are often viewed with skepticism. Recently, however, some well-publicized evidence of scientific support for folk beliefs has led to somewhat greater receptivity to alternative ideas. Consider the example of chicken soup, long a staple in the folk arsenal of cold remedies, which scientists have confirmed is a valuable intervention. In fact, there is growing evidence that interaction among belief systems may produce excellent outcomes as long as the several perspectives involved are valued. In *The Scalpel and the Silver Bear* (1999), Alvord and Van Pelt describe the ways in which Alvord, a Navajo surgeon, used traditional Navajo healing to provide psychological comfort and encouragement at the same time that surgical interventions were providing a physical "cure."

Another example of this kind of emerging scientific support for long-held folk beliefs is the growing body of literature about the **placebo effect**. By definition, placebos are inert substances or procedures. In many drug studies, participants are given either the "active" drug or a placebo, typically a sugar pill. In study after study, results report that the drug was either more effective than the placebo or no more effective than the placebo (Bernstein, 1999; Blakeslee, 1998). Over time, thoughtful observers have noted that although it would be expected that an inert substance would not affect the illness, in most studies some people showed therapeutic effects while taking the placebo. This finding was quite consistent. For example, a study might show that in both experimental and control groups, 10% of participants improved, or that 15% of control patients and 20% of participants in the experimental group showed improvement. How could this be explained if the control group was given an inert substance? Researchers were intrigued, and an array of studies has now demonstrated that the placebo effect is a potentially potent treatment option.

Adding weight to this finding are studies of so-called placebo surgery (Stolberg, 1999). Studies of brain surgery for Parkinson's disease have compared actual surgery with a procedure in which an incision was made into the head without further intervention in the brain. Other studies are examining arthroscopic surgery, comparing surgical procedures that scrape cartilage with procedures that simply make an incision. In these and other controlled experiments, placebo surgery has proved effective; in some instances, it has been as effective as the typical surgical procedure.

> ## MRS. CHEN
>
> Mrs. Chen, a 60-year-old Chinese woman, is brought by her daughter to a community mental health center. The daughter reports that Mrs. Chen has stopped going out and spends most of her time alone. The daughter, a second-generation Chinese-American, is concerned, as she herself is busy socially and fears her mother might be depressed.
>
> When the psychologist goes to the waiting room to get Mrs. Chen, her daughter stands up and walks toward the office with them. Both Mrs. Chen and the daughter seem startled when the psychologist suggests she needs to talk with Mrs. Chen privately. The daughter agrees, but with obvious reluctance.
>
> Mrs. Chen sits down when invited to do so by the psychologist and proceeds to tell the psychologist in a very soft voice that she has many stomachaches. She smiles frequently while explaining her stomach discomfort and looks mostly at her hands. She denies any other problems, although she then indicates that she is a bit worried about her granddaughter. Mrs. Chen seems reluctant to elaborate on her concerns.

These findings have puzzled practitioners whose frame of reference is strictly Western. How can they be explained? Perhaps any kind of intervention leads to an increase in endorphins, naturally occurring opioids that lead to a sense of well-being. Perhaps individuals who respond to placebos have personality disorders. Perhaps there are profound connections between the mind and the body that influence state of health.

This last assumption would make perfect sense to *curanderos*, acupuncturists, bonesetters, and shamans, all of whom believe that the body, the mind, and the spirit are inextricably linked. These healers believe that it is futile to treat only the body, without attention to other factors affecting well-being. They would hold that the placebo element is not inert but rather a powerful symbolic medicine based on belief and the strength of the human spirit.

However, a recent study (Hrobjartsson, Asbjorn, & Gotzsche, 2001) has challenged traditional thinking about the placebo effect. The two Danish researchers claim that while, in general, about a third of patients will improve if they are given a dummy pill and told it is real, participants given no treatment at all improve at about the same rate as patients given placebos. The researchers concluded that although placebos have no significant effects on objective outcomes, they have possible small benefits in studies with continuous subjective outcomes and for the treatment of pain. While this study calls traditional thinking about placebos into question, it will take additional studies to resolve this issue.

Clearly one dilemma is that it may be difficult to maintain objectivity in the face of the many different kinds of interventions and beliefs about cure. For example, it is not uncommon for some Asian and African individuals seen in Western clinics to have circular burn scars over their bodies. Staff have been known to report such individuals as being abused. However, an array of cultures use therapeutic burning, known as **moxabustion**, as a form of cure for such ailments as malaria, hepatitis, and abdominal problems (Feldman, 1995).

4-30. Think back to the last time you were sick. Can you identify any healing strategies you used (e.g., taking a bath, eating a chocolate bar) that made you feel better immediately but are not the kinds of strategies that might be suggested by a physician? What led you to try those strategies? Why do you think they helped?   **Q**

Clinical Encounters

Culture affects every interaction in the clinic. Understandings of health and illness; perceptions about effective healing; views about the relationship of the body, mind, and spirit; ideas about who holds authority in clinical encounters; and the roles of the patient and the healer are all influenced by culture. Divergent cultural influences exist even in relatively homogeneous communities.

Face-to-face interactions between provider and care recipient are most effective when they accommodate both parties' values about how they should be structured. Among the issues needing careful consideration are such factors as appropriate use of eye contact, understanding of views on privacy, attitudes about the body and acceptable touch, and personal space. In Western culture, direct eye contact is the norm. It is thought to indicate sincerity, interest, and connectedness. For individuals from some Asian cultures, direct eye contact is thought to be intrusive and rude. Many cultures have strong dictates about appropriate touch, particularly between genders. The idea of a male examining a female, providing a massage, or assisting with bodily functions would be extremely discomfiting to individuals from Islamic cultures, among others. Some cultures believe that information about one's body is personal, not to be shared. This attitude can be problematic in a Western-style clinic where it is considered normal to discuss body symptoms and function, often with a series of persons (e.g., an intake nurse, a physician's assistant, a medical doctor), all of them strangers. Culturally conditioned behaviors may interfere with the communication necessary even to determine the diagnosis. Consider the case of Mrs. Chen, described on page 74:

Q

4-31. Why do you think the daughter wants to come into the office with Mrs. Chen?

4-32. Why do you think Mrs. Chen might avoid looking at the psychologist? Why might she talk in such a soft voice? Does Mrs. Chen's smile mean that she is pleased? What else might it signify?

4-33. To deal effectively with this situation, the psychologist needs some specific cultural information, as well as more information about the symptoms Mrs. Chen might have. How can she or he go about getting that information?

4-34. What do you think Mrs. Chen believes is wrong with her? Do you think her daughter would be likely to agree? What about the psychologist?

Cultural beliefs are also found within professional cultures and can contribute to dilemmas in effective intervention. For example, the rehabilitation beliefs common among therapists in the 1950s and 1960s working with individuals recovering from polio reflected societal values. Clients were encouraged to be active and to exercise their muscles to restore strength. These beliefs shaped therapeutic interactions and seemed to result in positive outcomes in terms of regained function. More recently, however, a new syndrome—postpolio syndrome—has been identified in individuals who had polio and subsequent rehabilitation during the period. These individuals are now finding their rehabilitated muscles are failing them, and they are experiencing fatigue and functional deficits. The new wisdom is that the syndrome results from overuse of muscles, and professionals and clients alike are faced with reevaluating their firmly held beliefs about behavior and treatment. Rather than advising clients to stay active, therapists must now advise rest and relaxation, a recommendation that may be uncomfortable for both client and professional, if the older ideas about rehabilitation have not been erased (Scheer & Luborsky, 1991).

These cultural dicta about interaction are not immutable. For example, among Orthodox Jews, men and women do not touch individuals of the opposite sex except for their spouses and young children. However, cultural rules also allow for health exigencies to override this guideline. Thus, male physicians may touch female patients, both to examine them and to offer them comfort. In such situations, an Orthodox patient is likewise allowed to accept a touch that would be impermissible in another setting.

Culture and Health Outcomes

Positive outcomes can be defined in many ways. In Western culture, positive outcomes include cure of a specific illness, ability to undertake needed and desired activities, and self-perceived "feeling good." Until recently, medical practitioners perceived anything less than a total cure (i.e., absence of any biological disease process) as failure. There was a long period of time during which patients with terminal illnesses were shunned by such practitioners, and not until the groundbreaking work by the hospice movement and the writing of such authorities as Kubler-Ross (1968) was significant attention paid to **palliative care**—care to promote comfort rather than cure illness.

In other cultures, an important outcome is balance, even where an absolute cure is not achieved (Alvord & Van Pelt, 1999). Some individuals know at the end of a Navajo healing ritual (a "sing") that they are dying, but if they feel they have re-established balance with nature, they experience a level of psychological and spiritual comfort that might be identified as a positive result.

It is increasingly clear that one important factor in positive outcome is the belief the individual has in the treatment and the curer. In many cultures, the healer is in a special and somewhat separate group, held in high regard, not unlike traditional views of physicians in the West. Viewed as having a special calling, such curers carefully cultivate their image as a way to enhance their perceived abilities. In some of these cultures, it is considered inappropriate to inform patients of potential risks of treatment, as such information might create a mindset that would reduce the effectiveness of intervention (DiversityRx, 1997a). In Japan and many other cultures, practitioners avoid giving patients bad news—especially a prediction of death—for fear of the demoralizing effect of such information on the individual. In Hmong culture, predicting death is tantamount to wishing it on the individual. By contrast, special care is taken in the United States when disclosing side effects or potential risks in order to reduce claims of liability against practitioners. In fact, such disclosure is mandated by federal law.

Q   4-35. What are some potential consequences of the decision to reveal all possible side effects of a procedure to a client? Think about the discussion above of placebo effects. How might these be important in the process of full disclosure?

4-36. In your professional education, what instruction have you received about working with patients whose prognosis is terminal? Are you encouraged to discuss this matter with the patient? With his or her family? If you are not encouraged to do so, what has your education taught you about answering patient questions? On what philosophy about death do your professional guidelines seem to be based?

Organizational Culture in Health Care

As can be seen from the example of the Lees, organizational culture has a strong influence on practitioners and can come in conflict with beliefs of individuals seeking care. Organizations, like all cultural institutions, have rules. The rules dictate who may enter to seek care, who may support those receiving care, and who may provide care. They dictate how long and under what circumstances such individuals can stay, and they dictate behavioral expectations. In hospitals, patients are to receive care (ideally with appropriate gratitude), to

follow instructions, and to get better. Each care provider has a specific set of duties without deviation: physicians never change bed linens, and dieticians never tell patients their diagnoses. Behaviors that stray from the rules, no matter what the reason, often cause difficulty. A housekeeper who gives diagnostic or prognostic information may well provide misinformation and will certainly be disciplined. Families, too, can add to the dilemma by filling roles typically left to hospital staff. For example, among Korean families, it is common for members of the family to remain with the hospitalized patient at all times. Some may want to build small fires in the room to cook foods for the patient. Social support is clearly beneficial to health care outcomes, but most hospitals would see attempts to cook in the room as contravening policies and procedures.

The Western medical model is an authoritarian model that assumes that biomedical approaches work for everyone. This model casts doubt on most traditional health substances, such as herbs, and on other forms of healing, such as Navajo sings. Because it assumes that everyone has faith in biomedical approaches and in the providers of such care, alternatives are problematic. This stance is becoming somewhat more flexible as alternative models gain both popularity and research support, but it continues to be relatively rigid. One of the greatest problems with this stance, perhaps, is the likelihood that other methods will be denigrated. As already noted, a patient's faith in the healing method can be as important as the active effect of the method.

A particularly striking example of the problem relates to a case reported in 1957 (Blakeslee, 1998). A patient, Mr. Wright, had cancer and was given only days to live. He begged his physicians to give him injections of Krebiozen, a horse serum. They disapproved, but he obtained the medicine and immediately improved. His tumors disappeared and his energy returned. When Mr. Wright read a newspaper report 2 months later stating that the remedy was ineffective, he suffered an immediate relapse. Because of his previous improvement, his physician chose to reassure him about Krebiozen in spite of the physician's own reservations about the substance, and Mr. Wright improved a second time. Again, he read a report that Krebiozen was ineffective, and 2 days later he was dead. Mr. Wright might have died in any case, but this situation suggests that the rigid disapproval of treatments other than those accepted by Western medicine can have powerful effects.

Alternative medicine is gaining increasing

attention and respect in the United States. It has long been known that many Western medicines have their basis in herbal remedies. Other interventions such as acupuncture have existed for centuries in China and elsewhere. Regardless of the preferences of their physicians, many individuals are choosing to try such remedies, often with good results. The United States government has recognized the trend and established a National Center for Complementary and Alternative Medicine at the National Institutes of Health. The specific purpose of the Center is to study and evaluate a wide array of traditional and alternative health care strategies. Practitioners of such methods may be more flexible, but this is not always the case. *Curanderos* may interact comfortably with Western medicine, but other healers may feel that they must assert that their own methods are preferable. However, when alternative healers refuse to entertain the possibility that other strategies may work, they run the same risk as Western physicians of reducing the potentially valuable options available to the individual.

Health care encounters may emphasize cultural differences and exacerbate the potential for cultural conflict because the client is entering a new and unfamiliar cultural environment. The organization through which care is being provided has its own unique culture. A community health center will have very different values from a large tertiary care hospital, as both are finding to their dismay in this era of consolidation in health care. Within the health care organization, each professional with whom the individual interacts has not only a personal history but also a professional culture. A surgeon will undoubtedly have a different set of professional beliefs and values from those of an art therapist, and both may differ in their beliefs from those of the individual presenting for care. In addition, depending on the permanence and impact on the life of the care recipient, various illnesses, disabilities, and other conditions have their own cultures. A clear example is that of the deaf community, described eloquently by Oliver Sacks in *Seeing Voices* (1989). The deaf culture has, over time, experienced a number of severe conflicts with health care professionals. A well-known case concerns the debate around the use of sign language as opposed to instruction in speech and lip-reading. More recently, the use of **cochlear implants**, small transmitters that can carry sound waves in place of damaged nerves, has aroused controversy. As Sacks explains, the deaf community has a well-developed set of beliefs and values, one of which is the valuing of hearing-impaired children. Parents who are themselves hearing-impaired may be resistant to providing cochlear implants for their children, who might then be able to hear. From the parents' perspective, this intervention is destructive to their culture, whereas most health care professionals view the device as a miracle of modern technology.

Another example of the potential for problematic interaction between organizational and personal culture is in the expression of pain. Practitioners rely on reports from the individual to determine the kind of pain treatment required, so some individuals may be undertreated because professionals do not recognize the cultural factors that limit overt demonstration of discomfort. Likewise, in some health care situations, the "squeaky wheel" gets noticed. One woman described her experience in a recovery room following surgery. Raised in an undemonstrative family with a somewhat Calvinist ethic about expression of pain, she maintained a stoic silence even though she was experiencing both pain and a wish for reassurance about the procedure she had just undergone. A significant number of other individuals in the recovery room were from a much more vocal, expressive culture. These individuals were moaning, shouting, screaming their pain, and were receiving more attention from the nurses—attention that the woman wished she might also receive. Although in ordinary circumstances she recognized and respected cultural difference, in this unfamiliar, anxiety-producing, and medication-influenced situation she experienced considerable resentment about her treatment and about the behavior of the other people in the recovery room. On reflection after the event, she also indicated that although the nurses gave the other patients more attention, they seemed to exhibit behaviors (e.g., raised eyebrows, negative comments to each other) that suggested they likewise resented the patients whom they perceived as demanding. In this situation, the values, behavioral norms, expectations, and reactions of the woman, the majority of the patients, and the professional culture of the nurses were all in conflict, perhaps resulting in an unsatisfactory experience for everyone.

Another reason that health care encounters can be more problematic than everyday encounters is the fact that individuals entering the system for care often feel insecure and uncertain. They are surrounded by unfamiliar people and procedures, and are often separated from anything routine. Recall the last time you went to see your own physician. No matter how comfortable you are with health care environments, you almost certainly felt somewhat daunted by the setting. In such situations, people may lean heavily on established beliefs and behaviors as a way to feel some control over their circumstances. Given the tendency of health care providers to want to control situations, conflict is a probable consequence.

There are a number of areas of potential dissonance between patients and health care providers. According to the American Medical Student Association (1999), they include the following:

- Historical distrust. Many groups distrust the Western medical system. The Hmong, as we have seen, have a history that makes them suspicious of all perceived authority. African-Americans may also mistrust this system as a result of the experiences of African-American research subjects in unethical research studies—most notably, the syphilis studies in the southern United States in the 1930s and 1940s (Thomas & Quinn, 1991).

- Interpretations of disability. As we have established, cultural groups have differing views of physical change. What some perceive as disability, others may perceive as a special gift.

- Concepts of family structure and identity. Failure to identify the primary decision-maker accurately can lead to significant strife.

- Communication styles and views of professional roles. Differences in perceptions about the proper role of the provider are common and can lead to disagreement.

- Incompatibility of **explanatory models**. The Lees felt that Lia's illness was a result of evil spirits; the doctors suspected the improper firing of neurons.

- Disease without illness. A disease that causes no symptoms may not have a place in some cultures. Thus, high blood pressure, high cholesterol, and HIV infection may not be recognized as real entities.

- Illness without disease. In some cultures, a constellation of behaviors or experiences may be equated with disease, although for Western-trained practitioners, no disease is apparent. For example, a Puerto Rican mother might diagnose *empacho*, a stomach ailment she might describe as occurring because of food sticking to the inside of the stomach and causing pain.

One additional potential cause of conflict lies in health-seeking behavior. Brown (1998) describes a hierarchy for persons of non-Western backgrounds. Brown suggests that people have a particular order in which they seek care. Typically, the mother is the first line of care, possibly followed by a traditional healer of some sort, a pharmacist or other intermediate care provider, before a Western practitioner is consulted. Even for mainstream members of the Old American group—people who might think early of a licensed provider—consultation with a relative or friend may precede the trip to the doctor's office. By the time most persons approach a health professional, they have already probably tried home remedies and self-medication, informal consultation with friends and neighbors, and, perhaps, some alternative treatments. Whether for injury, for nonacute physical illness, or for mental health conditions, most patients have already formed a diagnostic premise, considered care alternatives, or even performed treatments. Almost no one enters a health care setting anxiety- or expectation-free, just as no one enters it culture-free.

Barriers to care are not all cultural, although cultural misunderstandings feature prominently among the reasons for failure to get health care (Ma, 2000). Other reasons include systemic issues, for example, the ease with which care can be accessed. Is it close to public transportation? In the immediate neighborhood? Socioeconomic issues also matter. What costs are associated with care? Can the individual afford the care? Does the individual know that sources of financial assistance are available? Is such help acceptable to the individual?

There is also the ever-present issue of language. Practitioners should bear in mind that language can be a problem even when both parties believe they are speaking the same one. A psychologist we know tells of the difficulties he had administering the vocabulary portion of a well-known intelligence test to a man who had grown up in an isolated area of North Carolina. The accents of the psychologist and the client were so different that they had serious difficulty understanding each other: one thought the word *bed* had a single syllable; the other, that it had two syllables, each including a prolonged "a."

4-37. Have you ever gotten advice about a health condition from someone other than a physician or nurse? Who was that person? How did you go about deciding whether or not to follow that person's advice?

4-38. Has a physician ever prescribed a treatment that you chose not to do (e.g., a drug you

Q

RESOURCES FOR FACTS ON CULTURAL BELIEFS ABOUT HEALTH

- The Center for Cross-Cultural Health (http://www.crosshealth.com/). A resource for links and videos.
- The Center for Multicultural and Multilingual Mental Health Services (http://www.mc-mlmhs.org/cultural.htm). Profiles of specific cultural groups.
- The Cross-Cultural Health Care Program (http://www.xculture.org/resource/library/index.cfm). Profiles of specific groups in the Seattle area but applicable to other areas; also includes a searchable library available to Seattle residents and has an excellent set of links.
- Cultural Competency in Medicine (http://www.amsa.org/programs/gpit/cultural.htm). Summarizes need for cultural competency and provides case studies of ethical issues.
- DiversityRx (http://www.DiversityRx.org/HTML/ESLANG.htm). Includes an introduction to diversity issues, links to other sites, lists of culture-bound syndromes, and theoretical articles.
- Ethnomed (http://healthlinks.washington.edu/clinical/ethnomed). Profiles of various ethnic communities; contains "clinical pearls" (brief descriptions on various clinical topics, such as circular burn scarring in Asian and African patients).
- The FIG Glossary (Brian Bell, 1996–1999) (http://www.eutopia.f2s.com/figit.htm). A handy table summarizing information about a number of folk illnesses, where the illness is found along with its description, links, and references.
- Health and Culture (http://health.csuohio.edu/healthculture). Resources, case studies, instructional materials, and opportunities to interact with others interested in cultural issues in health care.
- Indiana University Library Transcultural and Multicultural Health Links (http://www.lib.iun.indiana.edu/trannurs.htm). An excellent, comprehensive site for links to information about specific groups; also includes a comprehensive bibliography, some with Internet links.
- National Center for Cultural Competence (http://gucdc.georgetown.edu/cultural.html). Resources and policy briefs primarily focused on pediatric care; extensive bibliography of references about culture and health, with an emphasis on children and women.
- National Center for Education in Maternal Child Health (NCEMCH) (1999): Culturally Competent Services (materials from the NCEMCH Library) (http://www.ncemch.org). A comprehensive, annotated bibliography of references about culture and health, with an emphasis on children and women.
- Online Hispanic Health Resources (click on Hispanic Health) (http://www.library.uthscsa.edu/clin/resources/index.cfm). An array of resources related to health issues for Hispanic and Latino groups.
- Queensland Government (http://www.health.qld.gov.au/hssb/cultdiv/cultdiv/home.htm). An array of descriptions of cultural beliefs, emphasizing cultural groups prominent in Australia and New Zealand; includes bibliographies.

decided against taking)? Why did you choose against the treatment? How did you handle this decision with the physician? What were the consequences for your relationship with the physician? For the outcome of the health problem?

Implications for Health Care Providers

We have established that culture is important in people's everyday activities, values, and beliefs.

We have also established that health is a sphere in which culture has profound impact. For these reasons, care providers must be sensitive to cultural issues and be prepared to interact with clients in a fashion that effectively acknowledges and responds to those issues.

It is impossible to know every culture's beliefs. It is, likewise, impossible to know how those beliefs have changed as groups have intermingled and moved to new locations or how a single individual has modified, discarded, or adapted them. As can be seen from the example of hot and cold, subtle variations emerge over time and space, often in unpredictable ways. Practitioners must guard against making assumptions based on existing knowledge and must avoid overgeneralization and the use of broad labels—such as "Hispanic" or "Asian"—for a multitude of groups with beliefs that differ in small or substantial ways. In addition, as we have already noted, personal factors alter the ways in which an individual interprets information. Whereas generalizations about particular cultures provide a starting place, clinicians must identify the ways in which individuals have modified those beliefs as reflected in their own culture emergent.

Informing oneself about cultural beliefs can be valuable. However, having gathered information about a culture's beliefs, health providers must guard against prejudice and stereotyping that may be the result of inadequate information and inattention to context. There are many resources, including an array of on-line ones (see the box on page 79 for a listing of some of them), for gathering information. Particularly when dealing with something beyond one's experience, it is helpful to make use of these resources to gather basic information that can provide a starting point for exploration.

Q

4-39. Go to one of these websites and explore. Use the links to find additional information. Does your evaluation of the site correspond to ours?

4-40. Identify a specific health-related cultural belief. How might women and men or younger and older people interpret the belief differently?

4-41. Explain the cultural belief to a classmate or colleague. Discuss how you and she or he interpret that belief. Does it fit your world views? In what ways are your opinions the same or different?

A common problem is the potential for clashes of belief systems. A clinician might have to deal with the dilemma of a mother with a "hot–cold" belief system who does not give the proper dose of medication because she thinks it will produce "excess heat." In the example of the Lee family, the parents rejected medical advice that was inconsistent with their views on the best treatment and made determinations that they would not follow specific medication regimens.

Such behaviors lead to a perception of the client as noncompliant. This labeling is a particular problem in cross-cultural encounters, where clinicians are convinced that their interventions are right and good, and therefore essential. There are frequent news stories about individuals and families who decide to refuse surgery, reject blood transfusions or chemotherapy, or otherwise decide against mainstream professional advice. It is not unusual to hear of such families being taken to court to force treatment, especially when the patient is a minor and the parents are refusing treatment. Such confrontational strategies rarely yield satisfying results for either party.

An alternative strategy is being tried by some health care facilities that have chosen to examine their practices to make them more consistent with the beliefs of the groups they serve. For example, some hospitals are making use of **bloodless surgery** practices. These practices enable groups like Jehovah's Witnesses, who object to transfusions, to receive needed surgery. It is worth noting that hospitals using these practices have begun to employ them with all patients, because they are finding that the outcomes are better for everyone (Patrick Bray, personal communication, 2000).

Q

4-42. When you read or hear about cases where parents refuse to follow doctors' advice for their children, what is your typical reaction? Do you think that the state or other governmental agency should intervene to force the care?

4-43. Recall such cases as the parents' desire not to separate conjoined twins, even if one could survive. Can you imagine yourself in this situation? What would be your decision? Would there be any factors that might make your decision complicated?

4-44. Can you imagine the factors that might cause a person in that situation to make a decision different from your own? What is your opinion about a court decision that forces the physicians to separate the twins even over the parents' objections?

It is essential for professionals to recognize the potential for the validity of other beliefs. The previous discussion of placebos demonstrated that procedures discounted by the medical establishment may turn out to have some value. There is compelling evidence that faith in a procedure produces good effects, even when that procedure might not be consistent with what is recognized in Western medicine as best or standard practice. There is every reason to believe that non-Western interventions may have value, either because of the faith held in them or because of some real physiologic effect. It is important to remember that many currently accepted beliefs had their origins in folk medicine and that, over the years, many well-respected treatments have fallen by the wayside. Regardless of the clinician's acceptance of the potential validity of a treatment, the presence of that alternative within the client's cultural perspective requires the clinician to treat it respectfully and to seek accommodation.

Like the clinician, the client is juggling multiple cultural systems and trying to make sense of conflicting belief structures. Labeling resulting behavior as noncompliant suggests that the client is simply being difficult, rejecting what is obviously good advice. In fact, such behavior is rational and reasonable. It is the job of the professional to provide information in a form that can be used by the individual in making judgments and to help the individual evaluate that information in the context of his or her belief structure. Alvord and Van Pelt (1999) describe Alvord's experience filling in for a colleague on vacation and treating a patient of the colleague. A Navajo woman presented with symptoms of an inflamed gallbladder. Alvord felt that surgery was the appropriate treatment and convinced the patient to have the procedure, even though the patient did not feel the surgery fit her own belief structure. The patient died, and Alvord felt that this devastating outcome was a result of her insistence on a procedure or intervention in which the patient did not have confidence.

Ramifications for Health Care

What does all this mean for your practice? Clinicians in intercultural settings—that is, all settings—can start by approaching interaction with a particular mental orientation that acknowledges the complexity, multiplicity, and uniqueness of identities in interaction.

First, it is important to understand the complexity of interaction with individuals. Superficial knowledge of the individual's circumstances can never provide a complete picture of the situation. A diagnosis and demographic data provide only a starting place for information seeking.

Second, all individuals have multiple cultural identities, encompassing, for example, place or community of origin, current residence, religious affiliation, socioeconomic status, gender, and profession. By the time you have a full list of descriptors for an individual, you have probably described a completely unique person with a profile unlike anyone else. A 30-year-old Irish-American Protestant middle-class university professor may also be a weekend motorcyclist, making her different from any other Irish-American Protestant middle-class university professor you might meet.

Finally, regardless of cultural affiliations, personal factors will influence the individual's behavior and feelings. One must keep in mind that the client is a unique individual with a particular life history and background. Family dynamics, individual genetic heritage, and background all play a role in the beliefs and behaviors of individuals.

The health care provider must be attentive to an array of factors and must avoid the temptation to categorize and then treat the category instead of the client. At the same time, there are particular points of view in particular cultures, and these will affect the behavior of the individual as when cultural messages may encourage stoicism, behavior considered "histrionic" in Western cultures, or reticence. The health care provider can be most effective if she or he uses behavior as information and then attempts to determine the meaning of the behavior in the client's context. In the next several chapters, we describe in detail how you can go about accomplishing this goal in your own practice.

✎ Notes ✎

5

Recognizing Cultural Differences: Lessons from Ethnography

CHAPTER OBJECTIVES

By the end of this chapter, the reader will be able to:

1. Define ethnography.
2. Describe participant observation.
3. Describe how participant observation can be helpful in cross-cultural interactions.
4. Define vantage.
5. Discuss how position, values, assumptions, focus, and chance affect vantage.
6. Describe the application of the concept of vantage in cross-cultural interactions.
7. Describe and practice effective ethnographic skills, including questioning, keeping notes, seeing patterns, imagining alternatives, being prepared for surprises, attending to the individual and the group, and self-monitoring.
8. Define mutual cultural accommodation.
9. Describe how mutual cultural accommodation might operate in clinical encounters.

THE STORY OF LIA LEE

As Lia Lee's seizures continued, the mismatch in interpretation between the two cultures involved increased. From the Lees' perspective, Lia's doctors (as they categorized all the staff involved with the case) were not helping her. The Lees felt the medications were making Lia worse, and they were mistrustful of the doctors. From the staff perspective, the Lees were noncompliant. They felt that Lia, who was cosseted by the family, was spoiled and willful, and they increasingly dreaded the occasions on which the Lees would appear in the emergency room.

When Lia was 2 1/2, one of the physicians, using legally prescribed guidelines, decided that he needed to report the Lees to protective services on the basis of their "neglect." He believed that their failure to administer medications consistently constituted neglect as defined by law. After two hearings, both of which were confusing to the Lees, Lia was taken into a foster home. The Kordas, her foster parents, adhered rigidly to the medication schedule, but Lia's seizures increased.

The Lees were devastated and did not understand why Lia had been taken from them. After a month of total separation they were allowed to visit Lia, where the Kordas observed them to be excellent parents, deeply concerned about Lia. Nonetheless, if the Lees were not found to be fit parents within a year, they risked losing Lia permanently.

Over the period during which Lia was in their home, the Kordas came to know the Lees well. Foua came regularly to visit her daughter, and the Kordas observed their interaction. They themselves had difficulty with Lia occasionally and were impressed with the way in which Foua attended to her carefully and met her needs. In fact, they were so impressed with Foua's skills as a caregiver that they asked her to babysit for their own baby on several occasions.

Meanwhile, in another medical effort to reduce the seizures, Lia was placed on the drug Depakene. An easy drug to administer with few overt side effects, it had not been used previously because the physicians were concerned about its potential to cause liver damage. However, the Lees liked it because they could understand the simple administration instructions and felt it did not have negative side effects. Based on the Kordas' recommendation, they were finally permitted to take Lia home, stabilized on Depakene.

Lia's homecoming was celebrated with the sacrifice of a cow. The Lees believed that Lia had been returned home because foster care had made her sicker and that she was more damaged than when she had left. In addition to adhering to the Depakene regimen, they sucked the "pressure" out of Lia's body using a small cup heated with ashes against her skin. They pinched Lia to draw out evil winds. They gave Lia *tisanes* (brewed or steeped herbal liquids) made from herbs they were growing at the edge of the apartment parking lot. Although they were living on welfare, the Lees spent $1,000 on amulets with sacred herbs. As a means of drawing out the sickness, they rubbed a boiled egg yolk with a silver coin in its center, wrapped in a cloth, on Lia's body until the yolk turned black. Finally, they tried changing Lia's name briefly in an attempt to fool the *dab*.

The Lees also went to visit a *txiv neeb* (shaman) in Minnesota. They knew that *txiv neebs* believe that it is impossible to treat the body without treating the soul; the physicians had never mentioned the soul. This *txiv neeb* was thought to be very special, and so Nao Kao and other family members spent 3 days driving to Minnesota for the ceremony. The ceremony involved tying spirit-strings around Lia's wrist as had been done at birth. They also gave her medicine and performed other procedures.

Summarized from Fadiman, A. (1997). *The spirit catches you and you fall down.* New York: Noonday Press.

ETHNOGRAPHY AS A METHODOLOGY

Whenever you watch people doing something you do not quite understand and then reflect on what you have observed, you are using the basis of ethnographic methodology: close observation and inquiry. Ethnography is the study and detailed description of human groups using direct observation and interviews, among other research techniques. Ethnographic methodologies characterize field-based research programs in such disciplines as sociology, anthropology, political science, and public health. Ethnographic studies have been done of many small-scale societies in remote locations, but they have also been carried out among truck drivers, intravenous drug users, surgeons, and corporate managers in the United States.

Ethnographers gather their data directly, in a qualitative research approach known as **participant observation**. In this methodology, the ethnographer, or fieldworker, lives in a community and participates as much as possible in its routines. Constantly observing and always trying to behave as a member of the group, the participant observer is striving to derive the cultural system of the members on the basis of first-hand evidence and the evaluations received from the group. There is always more observation than real participation in these encounters, and true participant observation is a time-consuming and exhausting task.

Q 5-1. Think about your first experience as a professional in a clinical setting or as a student in a practicum course. How did you feel arriving for your first day? How did you learn what was expected of you not only in delivering service, but also in terms of social and professional behavior in that setting?

Ethnography, like other research models, has changed over the time it has been in use, and there are many good critical treatments of its implications and variations. We are not teaching ethnography here, but we do believe that some elements of ethnographic methods are the key to being able to implement the philosophy of this book in practical ways in cross-cultural therapeutic encounters. (A number of detailed accounts of ethnographic methods exist. Agar, 1996; Emerson, 1983; and Rossman & Ralls 1998 are good starting places for further reading.)

Several aspects of the ethnographic approach to understanding human behavior are directly relevant to the work of health care providers (Crabtree & Miller, 1999; Grbich, 1998; Spencer, Krefting, & Mattingly, 1993). First, we observe (or hear) something that does not make sense to us. Usually, this "not making sense" is the observer's problem, not the doer's. Unless there is some profound social or cultural dysfunction, the most likely hypothesis is that the doer's behavior is meaningful in some (cultural) framework that the observer does not share and thus cannot understand. The greater the difference in cultural backgrounds or assumptions between the observer and the doer, the greater the likelihood that they will not share common meanings about the behavior. Learning how the behavior "makes sense" is the task of an active, alert observer in a firsthand encounter with the life of the other person. In other words, it requires participant observation, a term that

> codes the assumption that the raw material of ethnographic research lies out there in the daily activities of the people you are interested in, and the only way to access those activities is to establish relationships with people, participate with them in what they do, and observe what is going on. (Agar, 1996, p. 31)

A second important feature of the ethnographic approach is the consistent working assumption that there is a point of view or context within which the behavior we observe (or hear about) makes sense and has coherence. That is, there is a framework within which the behavior is connected to other behaviors, values, and cultural assumptions within which it is meaningful and coherent. Agar's description of the task of the ethnographer is to figure out what that framework is, model it, and then confirm it through further observation and conversation. We believe the task of the health care provider using an ethnographic approach to understanding a client or patient is to assume coherence, seek a more elaborated understanding of the behavior in order to fit it into a context of meaning from the client's point of view, and use that context and point of view as aids to designing care and evaluating client behaviors.

Much of the time we all operate in contexts that are familiar to us. We pretty much understand the persons, interactional expectations, and behaviors we observe. We participate with others, using patterns of behavior that are usually unconsidered, patterns we may not even be aware of. When we interact with persons who do not share our contexts, assumptions, or patterns of interaction and behavior, our only entry point to understanding is careful observation, suspended judgment, and the assumption of internal coherence, even if we do not yet grasp its pattern ourselves. An ethnographic mindset is a strategy to help us maintain that mental perspective.

Some of the skills that make up an ethnographic mindset include the following:

- Empathy and good interpersonal skills
- Curiosity and the capacity for surprise
- Patience and a tolerance for ambiguity
- Reflexivity—the ability to self-reflect, observe oneself, and become self-conscious about one's motives, practices, and expectations
- Relativism—the suspension of judgments and evaluations based on one's own cultural systems
- Intellectual humility—the awareness of gaps in one's knowledge and the limits of one's interpretation (Cerroni-Long, 2000).

These skills are in demand in every profession and can be acquired or enhanced through instruction, experience, and practice. Such skills are valuable in any therapeutic interaction, but are absolutely essential in those involving intercultural interactions.

Q   5-2.   Again, think about your first clinical experience or practicum. What was your supervisor like? Did your supervisor do specific things that helped you learn the expectations of the situation? What were those things and why did they help?

5-3.   Did your supervisor do specific things that added to your discomfort? What were those things and why did they lead you to feel uncomfortable?

Cross-cultural interactions necessarily involve contrasts in experience, values, and assumptions about how to be in the world. Cross-cultural interactions in therapeutic settings add a further source of cultural contrast. There is the potential for specific and explicit differences in such central areas as the definitions and meanings of concepts such as health and wellness, sources of disease and illness, roles of care providers and sick persons, and proper behavior of participants in a health-related interaction. Because, as we saw earlier, each individual is a combination of physical, psychological, and cultural influences and experiences, any individual client

presents an almost infinite capacity for variability along these and other dimensions. Learning to listen carefully, observe closely, and interpret from within a broader context than the immediate interaction can strengthen your ability to enlist your patient's cooperation with diagnosis and treatment, ensure a more sensitive and caring environment for your patient's progress, and enhance the likelihood of successful outcomes. These skills can also contribute to your own sense of yourself as a health care provider, reducing frustration and bringing greater satisfaction to your interactions. In the remainder of this chapter, we introduce concepts and techniques designed to improve your skills at achieving an ethnographic approach to your work.

THE CONCEPT OF VANTAGE

Much of what is required to use an ethnographic methodology involves learning what to look for and how to see, record, and interpret what is observed. One extremely important factor in observing anything is the matter of vantage. (**Vantage**, as we use the term, was originally developed from a report of an examination of multiple perspectives in a monologue, later published [Hill & MacLaurey, 1995]. The concept has now been refined as the cornerstone of a theory of cognition [MacLaurey, 1997] but we adopt here only certain components of it.) Vantage is an element in point of view, in its most literal sense. Vantage refers to the fact that any observing mind has a specific point of view, and that point of view has physical, psychological, and cultural dimensions that restrict how much can be observed at any moment. Vantage is a concept infrequently talked about but always present and relevant. One's vantage always involves at least the following: position, values, assumptions, focus, and chance.

Position

Position is both physical and metaphorical.

5-4.   Look around the space you are in right now. What objects obscure your view?   **Q**

From where you are specifically located, only some parts of the space are visible to you. What is behind you is not visible at all. Of what you can see, some parts may be obscured by other presences in the space such as lamps, curtains, staircases, statuary, shadows, or fog. Your vantage is constrained by the direction in which you are looking, any obstructions in the area, and physical factors such as the direction of a light source or the weather.

You also carry a metaphorical positioning with you in any social circumstance, a position conveyed by gender and race, among other personal attributes, through the way you dress or speak, by your table manners, and in your title and the ornaments of your office. This positioning by status, role, occupation, wealth, and social rank puts boundaries on vantage by limiting both the ability to recognize aspects of another and the willingness to reveal aspects of the self. Positioning of both sorts, physical and metaphorical, is usually a given in any setting or interaction and is subject to relatively narrow possibilities of change. What is most crucial is to recognize that all observing eyes look from a specific position, and position informs and defines vantage, thus limiting what may be seen. All collections of data are therefore necessarily incomplete.

Q 5-5. What might reduce your ability to see what is happening with a specific client in the clinic? In addition to objects like chairs and walls, think about social characteristics of the space, such as the number of clients to whom you have to attend.

Values

Values, as discussed in Chapter 2, are also part of your vantage. Imagine yourself a vegetarian in a situation where meat is being butchered for food. How might your values in such a case condition what you see? How automatically or readily would your vegetarian perspective allow you to perceive the potential ceremonial and religious elements of the behavior and to value those independently? If you see a beggar, what values of yours are challenged or reinforced by that scene? As we have seen, our value orientation is part of our system of expectations and definitions. Value orientations control even such apparently simple domains as lunchtime choices.

As you determined in Chapter 4, various edible items may not be considered food in an individual culture. For most middle-class white Americans, for example, snake blood, horse meat, and roasted grubs are not considered appropriate for eating despite such potentially relevant factors as their ready availability, protein content, or flavor. Nevertheless, some Chinese people value snake blood as a remedy for failing eyesight, horse meat is a valued entrée in France, and roasted grubs are one of the few forms of animal protein readily available to certain nomadic groups in desert regions. Consider for a moment whether there are near relatives of these foods that are easily identifiable as food. What about duck's blood soup, venison, or grilled snails? These items are eaten by at least some middle-class Americans. Objectively, what makes one set of edible items food and the other not? Is not the determination of acceptability as food a consequence of value orientations—learning, cultural experience, and tradition—rather than some objective fact about the item itself?

When a devout Hindu accidentally and unknowingly eats something containing meat thinking it delicious, then vomits in disgust upon learning what it was, is that not a function of values overwhelming even physical senses?

Q 5-6. List a few specific items that might cause you to recoil in disgust if you were served them on a plate and expected to eat them with gusto. What values of yours do they challenge?

These values are part of vantage. They color our interpretations of what we see, and they may even limit what we can see. If we turn our heads in disgust, can we see everything?

Assumptions

All of us also bring a set of assumptions to every interaction. These assumptions include everything from what to wear to how to greet participants in the interaction, to what to talk about to how to react to a diagnosis, express pain, and follow health care instructions. When we watch an event or a performance, we activate a set of assumptions about its order, participants, and meaning. Such assumptions are part of our vantage. Each one eliminates some contradictory one, but each is built from our own experience, personal preference, and cultural training. If you attend an Indonesian gamelan orchestra performance expecting it to be like a performance of the Cleveland Orchestra, you will find yourself at a loss to understand what you see and hear. Your assumptions may limit your ability to understand or even see what the performers do and may keep you from appreciating the performance at all. Too long, too monotonous, too boring, you may conclude.

Q 5-7. Think about a time you went to a church service, party, or new store and found that your assumptions were not confirmed or your expectations were not met. What was your reaction?

Q 5-8. Now think about a clinical encounter in which you met a client or a health provider for the first time and formed an immediate impression (positive or negative) about the person's prognosis or competence. What led you to make the assumptions you did? In what ways did that initial guess influence your interaction with that person? In what ways might your assumptions have influenced the outcome of care?

To the extent that you conclude about some presenting patient that "those people are likely to...," your ability to see and understand has been compromised by the assumptions inherent in your vantage. We cannot eliminate assumptions, but we can become self-conscious and introspective about them and their role in constraining our vantage. We can challenge and change them, and remember that they are neither universal nor inevitable. We can suspend them for a time and learn to respect and even value alternative assumptions held by others.

Focus

Focus refers to the predetermined set of interests we bring to interactions. Focus enhances our ability to gather the information we need, solve problems, and complete tasks. It is part of vantage, and it provides order and priority to what we see, hear, acknowledge, and report. In doing so, it necessarily puts other things out of focus, making them irrelevant or even invisible. You can test this yourself any time you consult a television guide or a recipe, items we nearly always examine with a particular focus. If you are looking for a particular program to find out whether you have already seen this week's episode, how likely are you to notice that you have never seen tonight's episode of a different show? If you are trying to find a recipe for the leftover broccoli you have in the refrigerator, how likely will you be to read the instructions for making a new spinach casserole?

The same kind of focus orientation may cause a health care provider looking to diagnose a painful limb to listen specifically for physical symptoms and to be less likely to hear hints about psychological ones. A dietitian may be more alert to nutritional explanations, whereas a physical therapist is more likely to find a muscular one. Focus is essential to "getting the job done" and is always part of vantage. We may not be able to change focus, but we can learn to make explicit the ways in which it makes other information less salient in our view.

Chance

We seldom recognize the great role that simple chance plays in our daily lives. It is a significant part of vantage. We decide to observe this client at this moment and not another. We decide to skip this question and not another. A fire drill interrupts our interaction and we never pick up the disconnected thread of conversation, thus missing something that was intended to be said. The person we are chatting with is in the mood to tell a revealing story, and we have no idea what triggered that mood. From our vantage, the fact that we hear that particular story is pure chance. The unexpected encounter, the sudden juxtaposition of two objects, the new piece of information—any of these may bring us a new insight or interpretation, and all by accident. At any observing moment, we and our interacting companions have made chance choices that will constrain, however unimportantly, the content of our observations. The element of accident or chance always means that we did not see or hear other information or behavior. It creates gaps in our interpretations because it conditions our vantage (Figures 5-1 and 5-2).

Although all these factors may make it appear that our vantage is always inadequate, incomplete, and damaged, the fact is that we cannot ever be without a vantage. Everyone has to be someplace, has to be someone, has to have a past, and a task, and is in an incompletely controllable world. Everyone has a vantage. What is important to the ethnographic mindset and to good observational skills is to become aware of that fact and its implications. Vantage is what makes us humble about our interpretations because we are always aware of its potential to affect what we see and thus what we know or think we know. Once we understand the concept and power of vantage, we can acknowledge that others have a different vantage; that vantage can change moment by moment, through experience or learning; that we can make up for some vantage effects by using certain techniques; and that comparing information from different vantages is a practical and entertaining skill.

The experiences of individuals with Alzheimer's disease (AD) and their family members provide potent examples of the power of vantage. Alzheimer's is a progressive, incurable neurological disorder that causes increasing memory loss, confusion, and inability to perform common tasks. Currently available medical treatments are only marginally effective in slowing the progress of the disease. Individuals with the disease initially notice

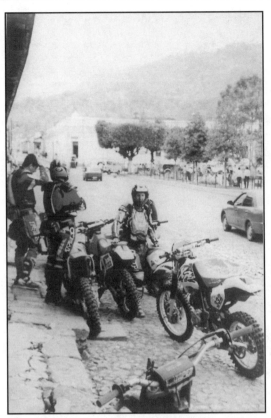

Figure 5-1. Motorcycles are part of the contemporary street scene in Antigua, Guatemala.

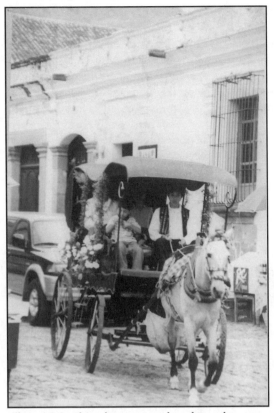

Figure 5-2. This photo was taken from the same corner, facing a different direction, seconds after the photo in Figure 5-1.

that they are more forgetful than usual. Perhaps they get lost in a familiar neighborhood or find themselves unable to do complex tasks at work. Family members may or may not notice these initial changes, because many individuals with AD are able to and want to mask these problems during the onset of the disease. As the disease progresses, however, the individual becomes increasingly incapacitated to such an extent that it is no longer possible to mask growing disability. Individuals who have written about the experience of Alzheimer's (Davis, 1989) uniformly indicate that these experiences are frightening and embarrassing. Such an individual may report, "I'm afraid I'm losing my mind." This is one vantage on the AD experience.

Meanwhile, family members indicate that before they recognized that the individual had a serious problem, they may have felt impatient and irritated with the person's inability to remember instructions and appointments or to accomplish simple tasks. They may have felt increasingly imposed upon by the needs of the increasingly dysfunctional person. They had another vantage.

Because of the media coverage of Alzheimer's and the diagnosis of such prominent individuals as former President Reagan, many people recognize the growing cognitive dysfunction as a problem and eventually seek medical care. Both individuals and their family members report a sense of relief when a diagnosis is finally made, despite the grave prognosis. The almost universal reaction is "I knew this was something real." Care providers, however, may experience the communication of the diagnosis as a wrenching experience. Knowing what individuals and families face, they may feel distressed at being the bearers of bad tidings. This is yet another vantage.

All of these experiences can create negative emotions, but there are other perspectives on the disease. Some individuals with Alzheimer's find themselves able to identify its positive aspects. They may feel surrounded by caring individuals and appreciative of the support provided. They may also frame some of the disease processes as giving them a new lease on life. One of us was meeting with a support group for newly diagnosed individuals in which one woman spoke of her delight at waking up one morning to see snow on the ground. Although snow was common where she lived, she could not remember seeing it before, and was excited about feeling it, tasting it, seeing it for the "first time." Likewise, family members often report positive feelings, particularly in terms of their pride at caring for a loved one and for being able to focus on what really matters in life.

Among professionals, some care providers advocate emphasizing these latter perspectives on AD (Fazio, Seman, & Stansell, 1999). They theorize that reframing the labels associated with an experience can reframe the experience itself. For example, they suggest relabeling anxiety as eagerness, agitation as energy, and wandering as exploring. A whole psychotherapeutic intervention strategy, rational–emotive therapy (Ellis & Harper, 1961), proposes the idea that much of human experience can be altered through reconceptualizing experience. We do not suggest that such relabeling is easy, nor that it always works. However, the discussion of relabeling reflects the fact that one's perspective or vantage influences one's perceptions of situations and events.

IMPLICATIONS OF AN ETHNOGRAPHIC APPROACH

Good ethnographic practice requires careful observation, close questioning, attention to vantage effects, and detailed note-taking. It rewards the practitioner by teaching or enhancing the capacity to develop and consider alternative observations and interpretations, heightening sensitivity and self monitoring in interaction, and building an awareness of pattern. The assumption of coherence is the assumption of pattern. Each observed behavior is assumed to be part of a larger scheme of behavioral patterns within which what is observed has meaning, relevance, and appropriateness. When we see someone who looks like us, talks like us, and generally appears to be a lot like us do something unfa-

EXERCISES TO BUILD CONSCIOUSNESS OF VANTAGE EFFECTS

- Spend some time with a young child in a place the child enjoys. Watch what the child watches, then talk with him or her about the shared experience. In all likelihood, your observations will be dissimilar to those of the child. Identify some of the aspects of vantage that constrain the way you see the child's world.

- Think back to the time when you were an adolescent. Think about an occasion when you and your parents disagreed about something you wanted, or did not want, to do. Can you reconstruct your parents' arguments? Your own? Now, from the vantage of adulthood and perhaps parenthood, can you identify some of the aspects of vantage that caused what your parents perceived as sage counsel to be seen by you as intrusiveness?

- Together with a classmate or colleague who seems much like you, choose a place to sit and observe for about 10 minutes. Choose a public place, perhaps outdoors, where people are engaging in various activities. The two of you should not sit in exactly the same spot nor talk to each other while you are observing, but you should be observing the same general scene. During your 10-minute observation, jot notes about what you see: where people are, what they do, what the surroundings are like. Also make a few notes about your interpretations of people's interactions. Then share your observations with your companion. Do your notes look the same as your companion's? What did she or he see that you did not? What elements of the environment captured your attention and your companion's? Were they the same elements? If you recorded observations of the same event, were your interpretations of its meaning the same? What are some other ways you might interpret the event? Try to account for the differences and similarities between your notes, observations, and interpretations in terms of vantage effects.

- Think about a time you handed in a classroom assignment or report of which you were very proud. Perhaps you felt you had a new insight or that you had gathered a number of important factual references. Perhaps you felt that you had pulled disparate information together effectively. What was your instructor's or supervisor's feedback on the assignment? How did you feel if the instructor agreed that it was very well done? How did you feel if he or she provided negative feedback?

miliar, it is relatively easy to assume that there must be something we do not know that makes the behavior make sense. When we see people who are not very much like us, perhaps with a different language or style of dress or way of moving their bodies, it is sometimes more difficult to imagine a context in which their behavior could be coherent. An ethnographic mindset gives us strategies for reminding ourselves that such a context is likely to exist and for helping us discover what it might be.

Attention to Vantage Effects

An essential component in such a mindset is the ability to see and watch out for **vantage effects**. Once you are alerted to the dimensions of vantage that we are highlighting here—position, values, assumptions, focus, and chance—you can easily learn to identify the ways in which vantage alters your own perception of reality. You must specifically call on your knowledge of vantage in order to develop the skills involved. Without specific consciousness, you are likely, like all of us, to perceive simply from your own vantage and ignore its effects.

In your own practice, you have or will have repeated opportunities to see vantage effects in action. Knowing about vantage and acknowledging its effects can allow you to appreciate varying points of view in new ways. Conflicts that appear to be about one thing may turn out to be about differences in vantage. For example, many clinicians have the experience of working hard to provide care for a particular patient. Perhaps it was a patient who had been difficult for others to care for. Perhaps it was a patient with an unusual problem. Typically, in such a situation, a therapist would expect the patient to express gratitude and a supervisor to give positive feedback. However, these responses are not always what happens. Sometimes the patient not only fails to express gratitude but actually complains about the care received. Sometimes supervisors, instead of valuing the care, criticize the excessive time commitment to a single patient. Rather than reflecting negatively on the care actually provided, such differing perspectives reflect different vantages on the same situation. The clinician has worked hard and wants appreciation, the client may feel overwhelmed and overworked, and the supervisor may be concerned about revenue generated. A clinician who is aware of the possibility of different vantages may observe the patient's facial expression and the supervisor's pacing, and recognize that the interaction is being experienced differently by the three players.

5-9. Review recent events or encounters in a clinical setting you have observed. How might this component of the ethnographic mindset contribute to better problem-solving or improved understanding in a workplace like yours?

5-10. Think for a moment about Lia and her family. How might attention to vantage have been useful for the care providers who worked with Lia? What are the fundamental differences in vantage that led to the claim of child neglect against her parents? What did the Kordas, Lia's foster parents, see that made them believe otherwise?

Careful Observation

Part of being human is the capacity to ignore or de-emphasize parts of incoming stimuli in order to concentrate on the parts that are considered more important or significant. Our brains are built to enable us to filter out large amounts of environmental data. If it were not so, we would be incapacitated by the sheer quantities of data competing for our attention. Some theories of autism suggest that lack of this cognitive filtering capacity is what creates the autistic mind and personality (S. L. Harris, 2000). The constant barrage of incoming stimuli, attacking every perceptual receptor, simply overwhelms the individual and produces strongly defensive reactions that serve to protect the exhausted recipient. As we build our filters and use our inborn cognitive capacity to assign some stimuli to nonessential status, we learn culturally how to select, how to make assumptions, and how to ignore elements within the array of data before us at any given moment. Once certain patterns are established, these ignored elements can become "out of awareness" to such a degree that we literally cannot and do not perceive them.

Recent research (Nisbett, Peng, Choie, & Norenzayan, 2001; Peng & Nisbett, 1999) has examined how the fundamental human cognitive capacity for categorization and perception is influenced by cultural factors. Comparative studies carried out in Japan, Korea, China, and the United States suggest profound differences between Asian and Western cognitive behavior in their descriptions of complex scenes with "focal" points and "background environment." These differences occur in such areas as scene-setting processes; statements of relationships between background and fore-ground; ability to identify focal elements against novel backgrounds; and tolerance for conflict, contradiction, and ambiguity.

Acquiring the capacity for careful observation in the sense we mean here allows us to cultivate consciousness and awareness about the environment of objects, persons, and actions. It means expanding the universe of data that we can perceive. It means learning to resort and recategorize in order to understand how persons with another learned filtering strategy might reorganize perceptions for purposes different from our own. Careful observation, the foundation of the ethnographic method, requires practice and some effort. Here is a sequence of activities to help you experience what such effort and practice is like.

Q 5-11. Go to a place you regularly visit or see and where there are always other people: a place on campus, your workplace, your place of worship, a neighborhood restaurant. Your assigned task is to "describe" a room or space in this familiar setting as completely as possible. Select a specific area you want to look at and sit comfortably and quietly for about 15 minutes, making brief descriptive notes to yourself. Include as much detail as you can. Then leave the place and let your notes rest for a day or two.

ETHNOGRAPHIC/ OBSERVATIONAL SKILLS

The key to ethnographic practice is observation. A number of very specific, practical, and learnable skills are essential for good observation: questioning, note-taking, pattern recognition, imagining alternatives, the capacity for surprise, attention to both the individual and the group, and self-reflection. In this section we provide some examples and exercises to help you learn and practice these useful skills.

We acknowledge that the emphasis in medicine on "getting a diagnosis" is often incongruent with ethnographic approaches to clinical care. Increasingly, however, health professionals are recognizing that a diagnosis does not provide a true understanding of client behavior. That can only come from the thoughtful use of ethnographic methods and perspectives. Even though a "diagnosis" may have explanatory power within the medical

model, it is not likely to be sufficient for the practitioner who seeks to provide culturally sensitive, client-centered care (Kleinman, 1980).

5-12. Review your notes from the observation exercise above. Recall that your instructions were to describe the space "as completely as possible." Here are some questions that will help you examine how well your description meets that standard. **Q**

5-13. Did you locate this space in relation to all the other buildings, rooms, or spaces in its neighborhood? Did you draw a map of the room or space itself to show all the items in relation to each other? Did you include a color description for each item in the space—all the furniture, the wallpaper, the clothing on any persons present, any equipment or tools you saw, books in the bookcases? Did you include noises, odors, the sensations of touch that you experienced while observing (e.g., your body against the surface on which you were sitting, a slight breeze from an open window, the temperature)? Does your description include size dimensions for the elements?

5-14. What is the item about which you gave the most detail? Would the detail in your notes allow you to describe it completely to someone who has never seen it? Using your description, could someone else build a scale model of the place or identify it in a group of very similar places?

5-15. How "complete" is your description? Where you could not answer the questions positively, can you account for why you did not include that information in your "complete description"? How did you feel as you read each question and realized that you had not noticed that aspect of the space?

Questioning

An essential observational or data-gathering skill is the ability to ask questions. Curiosity is a helpful trait in health care. Fortunately, health care practitioners work in settings where questioning is an appropriate activity. It is often helpful to assume from the outset that you do not understand everything that is going on and to ask for clarification. "How do you...?" "Why do you...?" can lead to clarification of beliefs, values, and practices, and confirm that understanding is shared. Too often, clinicians assume that they understand the other person's motivation when what they actually understand is their own motivation. There is the old joke about the woman who, when cooking, always cut her roast into two pieces before putting it into the oven. When asked by her mother why she did that, the woman said, "because that's the way you did it, so it must be right." The mother responded, "yes, but I only did it because my oven was too small for the whole thing." The younger woman could have saved herself trouble and the chore of cleaning a second roasting pan by asking her mother about the practice in the first place.

Q 5-16. Find a classmate or colleague with whom you feel you have a lot in common. Ask the person why he or she chose his or her profession. Try to obtain at least four reasons for the choice. Ask for clarification of the words the person uses. For example, if she or he says, "I want to help people," find out what is meant by "helping" people. Find out how the person will recognize when she or he has been helpful. How did the person decide that "helping" was what she or he wanted to do?

In Old American culture, there are many questions that are considered rude and inappropriate. One does not, for example, ask others about how much money they make (except in very specific settings such as job offer conversations). In other cultures, there are also areas that are not considered appropriate for questioning. For example, in Mayan culture and many Islamic groups, there is reticence about discussing sexual activities. However, in the clinic, some of this information may be central to therapy. In such cases, it can be helpful to ask first whether one may ask: "I need to know about X in order to help you. May I ask you some questions about X, or would you prefer not to talk about it?" You may also give the individual the option of talking to someone else, perhaps someone of the same gender or closer in age to the client, as both gender and age differences between clinician and client can lead to heightened reticence. A client who prefers not to discuss a subject may feel more comfortable as she or he gets to know you better or if you provide a clear explanation of why you need to know that particular information. Another alternative is to ask the patient if you can talk with a family member. Close observation may yield the information if con-

versation does not. It is often possible to find ways to design interventions even if you are missing some relevant piece of information.

Q 5-17. Think about a health care interaction in which you were the client and in which you were asked embarrassing questions. How did you feel? How did you behave? How fully did you answer?

5-18. Now think about an occasion where you were the practitioner (or observing a practitioner) who asked sensitive questions of a client. Were you hesitant to ask, or did you observe hesitation on the practitioner's part? What were the signs that made you realize that the line of questioning was a sensitive one? Did you think the client answered fully? What efforts were made to make the client more comfortable?

Some questions may be culturally off-limits, but individuals also construct areas in which they are more or less reticent that may have to do with personal experience and personality preferences rather than cultural factors. For example, one woman we know prefers never to discuss her family. No one knows why, but information such as how many siblings she has or where her parents live, which other people share readily, is sensitive for her. It is not possible to be aware of all of these individual differences, but it is possible to be cautious and observant when questioning. Respect for a client's preferences cannot keep us from gathering the information we need to do our jobs, but an awareness that questions may be unexpectedly sensitive helps us look for ways to explain why the information is needed or to provide contexts in which it might be more easily provided. Would the client prefer to complete a form rather than talk through it? Would sharing a little personal information of one's own make the information-gathering easier? Would a display of curiosity and openness about a range of factors in a client's experience and not just the presenting condition build better rapport and confidence? Ethnographic questioning proceeds on a case-by-case, moment-by-moment agenda.

Q 5-19. Review a common diagnostic or medical history questionnaire used in your discipline. Can you identify questions that are more or less invasive?

Q 5-20. Are there any questions that a typical Old American client might have trouble with? Can you find some questionnaires used in your discipline that assume an Old American cultural background and thus may be problematic for someone of another cultural history? How might those questions be prepared or rephrased to make eliciting the information easier?

5-21. List some of the questions you think were not asked in the case of Lia and her family that ought to have been.

Note-Taking

Getting the data is only the first step. We also must be able to record the data we observe and the answers we obtain. Therefore, we need note-taking skills. Each individual has particular habits with regard to note-taking, and some professions teach discipline-specific methods as well.

Q 5-22. Compare some of your class or meeting notes with those of one or two other students or participants to get a sense of how much your own note-taking style varies from those used by others.

Despite these differences, it is always important to make sure that notes include at least the following basic information: date and time of day (at beginning and end of session), exact location, persons present and their occupations or relationships to each other, language used, and purpose of the gathering. A small diagram of people's locations and perhaps a set of numbers or initials to identify each one may be helpful. Be sure to number the pages.

After the context for the notes is established, note-taking can begin. As you have learned from previous exercises in this chapter, it is not always possible to know in advance what will be important and what can safely be ignored. It is therefore important to cultivate good memory skills, abbreviations that increase speed, and the ability to record as much information as possible. It is also important that your notes consist of facts and direct observations, not of your own interpretations. For example, you might record that a person avoided direct eye contact or looked away while a particular topic was discussed, but you should not record that the person "looked shifty" or "was being deferential" or "was lying." You must keep notes on your own reactions

and on your interpretations of the interactions, but those notes should be separate and clearly identified as interpretive, not observational.

Good notes usually require a little extra time after an encounter is concluded. You might need to fill in information that was left incomplete. You might need to clean up unintelligible writing or abbreviations while you can still recall the content. Making these repairs soon after the encounter permits you to have greater confidence in your observations and, over time, may even improve your capacity both for observation and for note-taking.

At this point you can evaluate and interpret your notes. Make additional notes now about new or unanswered questions. Identify all points at which additional information is needed. This process of expansion builds on your current notes and prepares you for future encounters. Record any advice you gave or questions the individual asked. Do this review as soon as you can after the interaction is over, because your short-term memory will eliminate all "nonessential" data before long. Now is also when you should reflect on the interaction and critique your own questioning, observational, and interactional acts. Are there patterns of which you should be aware? Are there behaviors you want to change?

5-23. Return to your notes from question 5-11. Read them carefully to analyze and evaluate them. Can you see patterns in the way you describe objects? **Q**

Many people describe objects based on the function they imagine for them. Others focus on size, shape, or color. Others speculate about the materials from which they are constructed or on their positional relation to other objects in the vicinity.

5-24. On what types of data do you seem to be inclined to focus? **Q**

People also differ in the way they describe people. Some provide physical descriptions—height, weight, skin color, hair texture, clothing, posture—and others give more attention to behavioral attributes such as facial expression, gestures, apparent mood, or goal. What types of information seem to be easiest for you to observe?

Reconsider your description in light of the various questions asked earlier.

Q 5-25. Think about why the various types of data you did not notice or include were omitted. Did the omissions result from the effects of your vantage? Might someone with less familiarity with the scene have observed more?

Look for opportunities to practice this sort of observation, note-taking, and evaluation activity. You can practice note-taking by listening to a radio or television talk show, for example, or at a family dinner table conversation, or while in a meeting where you would not normally take many notes. Do not stop with the note-taking itself. Include in your practice the processes of review, repair, evaluation, interpretation, expansion, and self-critique. Seek opportunities to compare your notes with those of others. The more examples you can see and the more practice you can get, the better for your own developing skills.

Q 5-26. Again, find a partner with whom to discuss your professional interests and choices. Talk together for a few minutes in comfortable surroundings about your reasons for selecting the profession. This time, try to work with someone who is likely to have life experiences that are much different from yours (e.g., someone older or younger than you, from a different part of the city or country, or from a different cultural, ethnic, or religious background). Asking each other questions, talk with your classmate or colleague about his or her reasons for choosing a professional discipline and about the experiences or interests that led to that decision. While chatting, keep careful notes. As much as possible, record the exact words using a shorthand code if necessary. Sketch the person's posture and note any changes. Record the person's tone of voice and any changes as he or she talks. In your notes, indicate when the posture and voice changes occurred. Record facts and observations, but do not make any interpretations. For example, note the person's skin tone and changes in it ("during our conversation about X, her skin became more pink"), rather than making inferences ("she looked embarrassed"). When you have finished chatting (no more than 5 or 10 minutes), take a few moments to review and complete your notes.

5-27. Now share your recorded information with your partner. Does he or she agree that you

captured what was said? Did he or she capture your comments accurately, in your opinion? Where are the inaccuracies or differences of perspective? Are there patterns in the inaccuracies? What suggestions can you or your partner make to each other that will improve your note-taking skills over time?

Pattern Recognition

Good ethnographers develop abilities both to see pattern and to imagine alternative organizations, meanings, or interpretations. Using your notes from the two interviews about professional choice, you may be able to see patterns in the ways individuals decide to become occupational therapists or psychologists or nurses. For example, we know that people make career choices because of personal familiarity with the field, perhaps because a family member worked in that profession or the individual received service from someone in the profession. People may have other, less common reasons as well.

5-28. You now have three sets of data from your two classmates or colleagues and yourself. What are the main reasons why you three decided to go into therapeutic professions? If you are all in the same one, what specific reasons seem to be related to that choice as opposed to some other health field career choice? Prepare a list of common reasons for the choices made by people in your group. **Q**

5-29. Share your list with your class or group and listen as they share theirs. Together, determine the main reasons that people chose the various health-related professions reflected in your group. Discuss your findings until the group reaches a consensus about those reasons.

5-30. Now, identify the rationales that seem the most uncommon or unusual. Generate some theories about the shared reasons, as well as the uncommon ones. How common is the "personal familiarity" reason in your group? It is somewhat unusual for an individual to be unable or unwilling to give a reason, but perhaps someone in your group did not. Why might this be? Why is it important to examine findings that do not fit the pattern?

Humans are designed to see pattern and to act on it. An old saying suggests that "once is a trend, twice is a habit, and three times is the way things are." What this saying underscores is the human propensity for seeing pattern—if it happens twice, it must be a pattern—and for expanding patterns to assume they are universal. If we did not have this capacity, we could not learn. Everything around us would seem random and disconnected. Our brains strive to find pattern, even in stimuli that are not inherently patterned, as when we begin to assign stresses and beats to random tones or when we see familiar images in random water ripples or clouds or the brush strokes on a ceiling. That tendency then leads us to ignore what does not fit the pattern. The ethnographic mindset calls for us to pay attention precisely to the elements that do not fit, as they often serve as evidence that we do not yet accurately see the pattern but just parts of it. It is almost always useful, no matter how sure you are that you understand why someone behaves the way he or she does, to spend a little time thinking about **alternative explanations**, trying to see a different pattern.

Imagining Alternatives

Imagining alternate explanations is somewhat like that old child's game: How many uses can you think of for a brick, or an iron, or an earmuff? Stretching your ability to imagine even outlandish uses—An earmuff as a corsage? An iron as a paperweight? A brick as a water filter?—is good mental practice for the more serious work of being open to the effects of vantage on your ability to see pattern and meaning in the behavior of others.

The ability to imagine such variation leads to what has been termed **multiple subjectivities** in therapeutic encounters (Rakos, 1999), or the interaction of multiple explanatory vantages. The ability to imagine alternatives can facilitate understanding of alternative perspectives, enhancing empathic response.

The Capacity for Surprise

All these ethnographic skills are enhanced by cultivating the ability to be surprised. What we mean by the **capacity for surprise** is simply a men-

MULTIPLE SUBJECTIVITIES

Psychotherapists must recognize that "being objective" is not the goal in working with a client, and is probably not possible. Instead, the therapist recognizes that in every interaction a range of **alternative interpretations**, or multiple subjectivities, exists. Particularly in the early stages of therapy, this recognition provides the foundation for a therapist to communicate nonjudgmental acceptance and empathic understanding to a client, even if the therapist harbors a belief that the client is adhering to an idiosyncratic or nonconsensual interpretation of the event. The differences between the therapist's (and perhaps society's) interpretation and the client's interpretation frequently involve conflicts in values, but the employment of multiple subjectivities by the therapist allows the therapist to build or solidify the therapeutic relationship and defer clinically necessary challenges or confrontations until a time when the relationship is strong enough to withstand such stressors.

For example, a client may begin a discussion of marital discord by describing his partner's constant negativity, criticism, and public sarcasm. It quickly becomes apparent to the clinician that the client is very controlling and emotionally withdrawn from his partner. The client, however, views his style as masculine, similar to the behavior exhibited by his "buddies," and nonproblematic. From the therapist's perspective, this client's values are sexist and dysfunctional in the modern environment. Personally, the therapist finds the client's values offensive. Nevertheless, by adopting multiple subjectivities, the therapist is able to understand, accept, and empathize with the client and develop the sound relationship that may permit constructive therapeutic intervention. Such a relationship may over time provide the therapist with opportunities to share his own views and to encourage the client to consider the damage he does to himself and others by his negative attitudes toward women.

Rakos, R. (1999, May). *Control and countercontrol in the therapeutic relationship: Ethical and legal issues for behavioral clinicians.* Presented at the annual convention of the Association for Behavior Analysts, Chicago, IL.

CULTIVATING SURPRISE

A psychologist described working with a woman who had been diagnosed with schizophrenia. The woman, then age 27, had been in and out of psychiatric facilities and psychotherapy since age 17. She had been on a wide array of psychotropic medications over the years, none of which had been effective. She reported hearing voices and was agitated and unkempt. The psychologist suspected that the prognosis for the woman was poor because so many efforts at intervention had failed. The psychologist decided to try to get as much information as possible about prior events in the hope that there might be a clue somewhere as to how she might approach therapy with the woman. Simply because she was curious, she asked the woman to provide a physical description of her current appearance. She also asked numerous questions about the woman's feelings about being in the hospital and her conception of herself as a self-described "mental patient." In the course of the questioning, it emerged that the woman could not provide a detailed self-portrait, nor could she see any alternate self-portraits. Over time, the therapist encouraged her to develop a picture of herself and an array of alternate portraits, and to develop them fully. To the therapist's surprise, one day the woman said, "The picture I like best is of being just like you. I'm tired of being a patient." At that moment, a significant turnaround occurred, and 4 years later, the woman was out of the hospital, off medications, and pursuing a doctorate in psychology.

tal readiness to learn that one's tentative interpretation is incomplete or incorrect. It is the process of accepting, not simply disregarding, contradictory information. Whenever you think you know what is going on or what something means, you may limit your ability to process a contradictory piece of information or to imagine a different explanation. Being prepared to be surprised means being prepared to adapt your interpretations and interventions to new observations.

Q 5-31. Read "Cultivating Surprise" above. What was most surprising to you in the example of the psychologist and the supposed patient with schizophrenia?

5-32. Can you recall an occasion where your assumptions and interpretations were challenged by observation or when you were surprised to learn that you had been wrong? In thinking about this occasion, can you recall the moment when you realized your error and arrived at the new interpretation? How did you feel?

Attending to Both the Individual and the Group

Another aid to enhancing your observational abilities is learning to attend to the individual as well as to the group. Obviously, if you know that a person was born in Japan of Japanese parents, you can make some assumptions about what the person is like. The more you know about Japanese culture, the more you may recognize as Japanese in the person's dress or language or manner. You may be able to build rapport more quickly, using your knowledge of Japan and its culture as a foundation. The more you know about the different cultures represented among those with whom you interact, the better. However, any individual person is not "the Japanese" but rather "a person who, among other things, is Japanese." Thus, factual knowledge about a particular country or culture is not enough, especially if that knowledge is gleaned primarily from tourist or stereotypical sources. It is essential to keep focus on the individual, not on group stereotypes.

A common example of an over-large category label that obscures important differences that distinguish internal groups and individuals is the term "Hispanic" (or its close relatives "Latin" and "Latino"). Originally meant to refer to cultures or groups that derive from the Iberian Peninsula, it is widely applied to persons from a large geographic area extending from the southwestern United States through Mexico and Central America, and across all of Latin America, including Brazil, plus some Spanish-speaking islands of the Caribbean. In common use these days among people interested in multicultural issues of education, the label is occasionally used in phrases such as "the Hispanic way" (Nobel & Lacasa, 1991) or "in the Hispanic culture" (Cuellar & Arnold, 1988), suggesting that persons from the large region inevitably share cultural norms or ways of behaving or even thinking. However, each individual country in the region has a unique history, with unique sets of cultural influences and contacts and very diverse internal populations. Brazil is often omitted from the category, precisely because its historical experience of language (Portuguese, not Spanish, is the dominant language), colonialism, immigration, race, and economics, among much else, has been unlike that of its neighbors in South America. In addition, each country differs in size and geography, time and type of European contact, natural resource availability, post-independence political history, and relations to other nations. All these factors contribute to individual "national" cultures.

Across the rest of South America, varieties of the Spanish language differ from one region to another. Depending on such factors as the level of education an individual has and how familiar he or she is with other Spanish language groups, two varieties of Spanish may even be mutually unintelligible. That is, uneducated Spanish speakers from very different backgrounds may not understand each other because of differences in pronunciation or vocabulary. Moreover, many of these countries have large indigenous populations whose impact on cultural forms and even language has been extensive. It is simply not possible to know, in advance of interacting with an individual from one of these places,

how much he or she might resemble some pre-existing notion of how Hispanic people think or behave. (By now, you should realize that the very notion of a culture-wide or geographically based "way of thinking" is a fairly useless idea anyway.)

Even within a single group, such as Venezuelans, there are many possible subgroups with varying ways of behaving and differing cultural concepts. Men who are native to the undeveloped plains, or *llanos*, region of southwestern Venezuela, for example, have a long horse-based, self-reliant, family-oriented cultural tradition that is associated with notions of ruggedness, rebellion, and close ties to the land. The 19th century hero Simón Bolívar, the great liberator of Venezuela and other South American countries, came from this region. The tales of his military leadership and success against the colonial Spanish government are part of a strong regional sense of history. The cowboy-like traditions there resemble those of the American West much more than they do the Caribbean- and African-influenced cultures of the Venezuelan coast or the northern highland regions with their tremendous level of contact with descendants of the Andean Inca or the lowland Amazonian rainforest regions of the southeast. An *llanero* professional who has studied in a highland university and now works in a computer start-up in the coastal capital of Caracas and takes adventure

THE PERSONAL AND THE CULTURAL

Hashimoto (1996) did an extensive ethnographic study of four women, two American and two Japanese, older than age 60. Among the issues explored were social support networks and activities. Here are some quotes from the women:

"I do nothing. There's nothing to do here. I haven't got none, no friends.... On a Sunday, the parking lot is full when they come to see their grandmother or their mother, but there's nobody there for me...." (p. 1)

"I do nothing all day. I used to like making cloth flowers. I gave them away, but I ran out of people to give them to; so, I don't do it anymore." (p. 3)

- Identify which of these statements was made by the Japanese woman and which by the American woman.

The first statement is by Dorothy, an American woman, and the other is by Shizu, who is Japanese. Both of these women feel they have nothing to live for. Dorothy lives in a small, subsidized housing unit, supported by Social Security. She has arthritis, which makes it difficult for her to get around, and her husband and two daughters have died. Her son had a stroke and is paralyzed. Shizu lives in a rental unit with her husband. She also has arthritis and moves with difficulty. In keeping with Japanese tradition, Shizu has adopted a nephew and niece as adults to provide support for her in her old age. However, although she acknowledges that they are very good to

continued

her, she says she does not want to trouble them, and even with this apparent support network she feels alienated.

The other two women describe their lives quite differently. Irene, a retired school teacher, sees herself as primarily a provider of support to other elderly individuals. She is still married but has no children of her own. Suzuki is a nurse in her late 60s who is still professionally active. She has a mild hearing problem, is widowed, and has three children who live in other cities.

"Most weeks, I'm out of the house every day for some part of the day.... I believe that growing old is part of growing. It's the continuum of life.... In order to be alive, I had to be involved."

"There's so much to do all day. I haven't got any quiet time for myself, oh really... I've got so much to do!"

- Can you tell which of these is Irene and which is Suzuki?

The first woman is Japanese and the second is American. Although living in very different communities, Irene and Suzuki have more in common than Irene and Dorothy. Suzuki has more in common with Irene than Shizu.

---

vacations on the Amazon River surely does not share the world view, experience base, or value system of his *llanero* brother who took over the family farm. As in the United States, regional differences in other countries also produce cultural identities (e.g., westerners, southerners, "rustbelt" urbanites, "beltway insiders") that may be overlays or substrates for additional occupational, ethnic, religious, and other identities.

It is important not to underestimate the possible influence of such differences in individual experience as travel, broad reading, or education on cultural values or ideas. All these opportunities to extend beyond our own local boundaries change the informational base and potentially the world view within which we operate emotionally, intellectually, and even physically. Being exposed to yoga, for example, can affect our perceptions of the cultural values related to work and spirituality and alter our notions of stress and health, even though it does not turn us into Indians, Buddhists, or New Agers.

Q   5-33. Think about your own life. Has travel, educational experience, or a particular book influenced you in significant ways? Made you change your views on some topic? Given you an alternative understanding of part of your world? Brought new elements to your cooking, your home decor, your leisure activities, your dress, your ideas about God, your political views?

These same experiences have the same types of effects on other people as well, so it is just as well not to indulge in superficial categorization of other individuals on the basis of simple sets of cultural

generalizations. Though it may be possible to create great generalizations in broad strokes about the way a large regional or national group thinks about politics, the environment, or any topic, it is generally useless to rely on them in individual interactions. Until you ask or learn about another individual's background, you cannot depend on any generalization to be made from such simple details as name or physiognomy or place of origin. The ethnographic technique is one of inquiry and cultivating curiosity, and the capacity to be intrigued by the individual. Check your own thinking on this point by reading and responding to the example in the preceding box.

Self-Monitoring and Self-Checking

Finally, an important component of progressive skills development in this field is self-checking—the practice of reflexive introspection, self-interrogation, and sharing interpretive observations with others who have a different vantage. Recalling that our data are always incomplete, that our vantage is always constrained, and that culture is always emergent should keep us skeptical about our judgments and analyses. However, we must act on what we have, just as a physician acts in an emergency room without complete data in hand. Sometimes we may have detailed information about some cultural "pattern," but the data may have been collected in only one setting that does not match the one we are in. Regardless, we must act. We have tasks to complete and patients to care for. Still, we also must engage in an ongoing practice of checking our hypotheses through more questioning or observation, by adding data and seeking alternative explanations, and by reconsidering and critiquing our own role and vantage. The practice of an ethnographic mindset is a lifelong endeavor, applicable to both professional and personal goals, and always susceptible to improvement and expansion. This final aid to developing these necessary skills simply means that once you have intellectually committed to this approach toward the therapeutic encounter, you can never get enough of it.

MUTUAL ACCOMMODATION

As we have seen, cultures are constantly changing as the individuals who shape them interact with each other or gain access to information from elsewhere in the group or outside. The contact among cultural groups is probably greater now than at any time in the past. In complex societies, especially, we encounter new artifacts, symbols, representatives, and ideas from other parts of our society almost routinely, sometimes on a daily basis.

Q

5-34. For one day, keep a log of all the contacts you have with other cultural groups, whether through conversation, reading (e.g., news reports, a novel set in a foreign country), visual media (e.g., a foreign film, advertisements for imported products), observation (e.g., visiting an international crafts store), or other sources (e.g., a new restaurant, a visit from distant relatives). Do not overlook groups with whom you interact often and closely (e.g., fellow workers, neighbors, or clients).

5-35. For each entry, consider and identify elements of that other cultural group to which you were exposed. For any entry involving information about other cultural ways of thinking or behaving, try to identify the contrasts they might pose to your own cultural training.

5-36. For one day, make note of the origins of items you have in daily use, such as clothing, food, or decorative materials. For any two or three items, consider the larger context in which they were created. Did you choose them over something more local? Why? What do you know about the geography, economy, history, or contemporary lives of the persons who make the items?

Culture Contact

Culture contact, the interaction of persons from different cultural backgrounds, can take place on a culture-wide scale or among a few individuals. Culture contact usually causes some type of culture change, often substantial, as when whole societies are disrupted because of such malign contact situations as conquest, war, or imported disease. Much has been written on the processes of culture change, and particularly on the process of assimilation, in which one culture, usually a subordinate one, adopts a considerable amount of another culture's goods and ideas. As one culture takes on the characteristics of another culture, it may be said to be assimilating those characteristics. Eventually, assimilation processes may result in the wholesale loss of cultural traditions through their substitution by new ones. These processes have affected, for example, many Native American groups, some of which are now attempting to reconstruct traditional religions, languages, economic practices, and other elements of their precontact cultures.

Deassimilation, the process of reviving cultural values and behaviors from an earlier time, is much more difficult than assimilation, often because the source information has been lost. For example, African-Americans attempting to revive the traditions of Africa may find it difficult to determine accurately what kinds of rituals and celebrations were undertaken by their ancestors or even where their ancestors came from.

Not all culture change results in culture loss or other negative outcomes, of course, and many groups are dedicated to managing culture contact and culture change in order to derive the greatest benefit from it. Health care provides an excellent example. There is no question that the addition of Western health care practices to those of other cultures can have beneficial effects on such health measures as infant mortality and longevity. At the same time, the addition of alternative and complementary practices such as meditation and herbal remedies has clearly enhanced satisfaction with Western medical practices for many individuals in the United States.

Remember that in Chapter 3 we mentioned the potential impact of Internet access in small, rural towns in Central America. This technological innovation represents the introduction of a dramatically different kind of culture into areas that have been relatively isolated over decades, even centuries. However, the introduction of this new cultural artifact may serve to save traditional culture by making local crafts more economically viable. New markets may open for these crafts where they can be sold worldwide, rather than just to tourists who happen into the villages. At the same time, access to these local crafts enriches other cultures, as potters share designs, for example. In this case, culture contact serves to enrich both rather than damage either.

Q 5-37. Consider more completely the example of Internet access in small rural communities in Central America. Together with a partner, make a list of three to five other possible positive outcomes of this contact and another list of three to five negative ones. Share your lists with other pairs and try to decide the likelihood of each outcome. Is there any possible relevance of the most likely positive and negative outcomes to your life in the United States?

Some types of culture change occur at a local level, as when new immigrant groups arrive in formerly homogeneous communities. For example, communities were changed when several hundred Guatemalan Mayans arrived in Indiantown, FL (Burns, 1993), or when Vietnamese immigrants settled in Houston, TX, or when several thousand Somalis were relocated to Columbus, OH. The impact on local human services providers, especially health care agencies, and on the educational system, religious institutions, and local economy can be rapid, powerful, and conflicted. These changes, even though they may be wide-ranging and permanent in the local area, may have relatively little impact on institutions at the county level, much less at the state or regional level. However, the effects within single agencies or offices can be substantial, and sometimes these environments present examples of what R. McKenna Brown calls mutual cultural accommodation (personal communication, 1999).

Mutual cultural accommodation is the process by which individuals make modest adaptations in their behavior based on new knowledge from a previous contact. The goal is to improve the interactional environment. The crucial feature is repeated association across cultural boundaries but not always with the same individuals. We have seen such accommodation in settings such as study abroad programs where new groups of students visit

the same host community, or in ongoing faculty exchange programs where different people from an institution visit another institution over a period of years, or in health clinics where various immigrant clients of the same background are treated by the same staff members. In these settings, communication with other members of the host site (a local home, a university department, or a clinic in these examples) can result in conscious changes in behavior on subsequent encounters.

Because these changes are largely conscious, we call them accommodations rather than thinking of them as examples of cultural assimilation. Accommodations do not necessarily mean that people are incorporating other cultures into their own, and they do not usually produce lasting or culturewide change. They are evidence of careful observation and strategic attempts at improved interaction. In health care settings, they can reflect a growing awareness of the power of culturally astute care to improve patient outcomes.

Such accommodations by care providers are not carried out in a vacuum because members of each community are also in communication with each other about prior experience. They may also alter expectations or behavior in ways that result from their analysis of what they observed or experienced before. For this reason, we refer to a process of mutual accommodation.

We have seen a good example in the case of a summer study abroad program in Guatemala where students from the United States visited Mayan households for discussions of traditional Mayan practices such as weaving or agriculture. During the visits, these students would share a festive meal with the family hosting the visit. Mayans typically eat only one large meal a day, and on festive occasions they serve special, labor-intensive dishes containing meat, for them a rare and expensive but very desirable food. A traditional Mayan meal is served on individual plates prepared in the kitchen. Also, Mayan etiquette dictates that food must not be left on the plate. As a common saying goes, "It's a sin not to finish your food." Unaccustomed to such large servings, finding the meat of poorer quality than at home, and unmindful of leaving what they did not care for, the students sometimes left large amounts of the meal uneaten. Some students, self-identified as vegetarians (a concept without much meaning among Guatemalan Mayans), would pointedly refuse to eat the meat dish at all. This situation caused considerable difficulty and embarrassment for the hosts.

MUTUAL CULTURAL ACCOMMODATION IN HEALTH CARE

If a client comes from a group that avoids eye contact with authority figures (e.g., Chinese or Vietnamese) and the provider comes from a group that highly values eye contact and expects it to occur during the session, a provider might wonder if the client is behaving normally. (A provider with a less ethnographically oriented mindset might simply conclude that the client is shifty and probably not telling the truth about symptoms.) Suppose she finds out from other providers that persons from that group typically do not make eye contact, and she also learns from their experience that things seem to go more smoothly if the provider does not keep staring at the client. The provider may well try to control and adapt her own behavior during the next interaction, even if that interaction is with a different person. She may try to speak with the client while looking away from her face. Meanwhile, the client may be advising a friend that at the health clinic people stare into your eyes and seem to like it if you stare back. Perhaps the friend will remember this advice when she next visits and will consciously try to make more eye contact. Each person in the interaction may be somewhat uncomfortable with these new behaviors and will no doubt be watching to see what, if any, impact they appear to have on the quality of the interaction.

Q 5-38. Before reading further, think about specific difficulties this situation might produce for the hosts. Make a few notes to respond to the following questions. What conclusions might they draw about food customs in the United States? What conclusions might they draw about the behaviors of the students? What questions might they ask of the study abroad program director in order to understand the situation better? What questions could the students have asked? How might the program director have prepared the students for this situation?

After a couple of summers, the host families began to change their way of presenting the food. Instead of serving from the kitchen, they began to put the food in large bowls, which they brought to the table, allowing the visitors to serve themselves. They also served the meat separately from the sauce and vegetables that accompanied it in the traditional recipe. These changes were not made at other Mayan meals; they only occurred when visitors from the United States came to the house. The first time or two, the hosts commented on the difference between this practice and their customary one.

Meanwhile, the students in subsequent summers were given more preparatory information about Mayan meal customs and etiquette. They knew they needed to finish all the food on their plates, and they understood more clearly the honor being done them by the serving of meat. Students

continued to highly value the sharing of meals with their Mayan hosts and expressed appreciation for the chance to select the items and amounts that suited them from among the components of the meal. Everyone seemed to be more pleased with the meal experience. Over time the hosts stopped commenting on the differences between the "traditional Mayan meal" advertised in the study abroad brochure and the accommodated version they were now serving. Students in later study abroad seasons did not even realize that there was any difference between their experience and that of earlier students.

5-39. Before reading further, think about the processes at work here. If the hosts had not accommodated in the serving of the meal, what accommodations might the students (or the study abroad director) have made to reduce the conflict between Mayan and typical American meal behavior? **Q**

5-40. Because the featured recipes were themselves the same and the overall types of conversations at the table were unchanged, were the study abroad students still experiencing "a traditional Mayan meal"?

Achieving Accommodation

Similar opportunities for mutual accommodation can occur in health care settings in the United

States as well. When a client of a particular cultural background visits a clinic, the care provider might consult with other providers who have interacted with clients from the same group. At a team meeting, the provider might share an observation or inquire about the experiences of the others in order to understand a behavior that seemed unusual. As a result of these conversations, the health professional might alter his or her own behavior to adapt to the client's cultural system. Meanwhile, the client might consult other family members or neighbors who also use the clinic in order to gain insight into the behavior of the provider or the processes of the clinic and, similarly, might alter behaviors to accommodate the provider. Consider the more detailed discussion in the box on page 102.

Such accommodations do not have to occur only when the interacting individuals are from drastically different cultural backgrounds. Consider the case of a psychologist we know whose first job was working as a mental health counselor with groups in a day treatment center in an inner-city, state-funded psychiatric hospital. The psychologist was a middle-class white suburban woman raised and trained in the midwestern United States. The treatment facility had a mostly African-American population, largely from the inner-city neighborhood surrounding the hospital. All of the clients had chronic psychiatric problems, mostly schizophrenia, and all had been in and out of hospitals for years. Clients were referred to day treatment from the inpatient ward and attended programs 5 days a week. The psychologist conceptualized the day treatment program as a bridge to "acceptable community reintegration." To her, this meant that patients would spend several months in treatment learning work and community life skills that would enable them to live independently in the community.

Over the first month, it became clear to her that although the patients came faithfully to the group sessions she organized, few attended to the content. In fact, she was dismayed to see that they often changed the subject, perhaps to discuss yesterday's soap opera on television, perhaps to gossip about the neighborhood. As time passed, it became clear to the psychologist that the patients had a very different view of the goals of day treatment. Most had never held jobs because of their psychiatric conditions. In the broader community, paid employment was not generally available to them. The patients enjoyed coming to day treatment as a social outlet and hoped to come for as long as they were permitted. Thus, the patients came to her groups as the "price" for being accepted into the day treat-

ment program but were uninterested in the substance she presented, as it did not conform to their goals.

Ultimately, the psychologist decided that helping the patients live without inpatient hospitalization was a goal that fit the patients' world view better than her own. A restructuring of the group sessions to focus on socialization was considerably more successful and, in the end, allowed several of the patients to make a gradual transition away from day treatment.

Typically, accommodation is taken to be the responsibility of the lower-ranking or less powerful individual in an encounter. You have probably noticed in our examples that even though we are speaking of mutual accommodations, the fact is that in most cases, the differentials in power, authority, and control cannot be totally obscured. It is important for an ethnographically skilled therapist to be alert to this dimension, which probably characterizes all therapeutic interactions to some extent.

The suggestion we make here is that providers can, and should, also exert themselves to accomplish accommodating adaptations when they expect to see several clients of similar backgrounds. We consider mutual cultural accommodation to be a positive factor in successful cross-cultural therapeutic interactions, but we also recognize that many of the perceptions that underlie them are somewhat off the mark. Because the process goes on mutually but independently, it is also possible for accommodations on one side to come up against contradictory accommodations on the other.

Despite these potential conundrums, however, we think the likely outcome of a well-established ethnographic mindset will naturally be the tendency to accommodate perceived differences in culturally derived assumptions and behaviors. Furthermore, we depend on the incorporation of ethnographically derived methods of observation to ameliorate the potential contradictions that may occur during accommodation. A self-monitoring, consciously reflexive, observant health provider with a routine practice of analysis, evaluation, and checking will be able to use mutual accommodation to the benefit of clients and to the advantage of his or her own developing ethnographic orientation.

5-41. Return to the place where you conducted your original observation exercise. Again, spend 15 minutes there, observing carefully. Do not make notes. Try to see everything equally. Become aware of your body and its sensations in the space. Try to bring to aware-

Q

ness just those kinds of data that you omitted earlier. After 15 minutes, spend a few more minutes reflecting on the experience of this exercise. What does the process of conscious awareness feel like? How different were your perceptions on the two occasions of observation?

5-42. What application might this multi-part exercise have to therapeutic practice? What behavior might the health care providers involved in Lia's case have observed that made them classify the family as noncompliant and the child as willful? What other behaviors might they have overlooked?

Q

✎ NOTES ✐

✎ Notes ✎

6

Negotiating Cultural Differences in Working with Clients

CHAPTER OBJECTIVES

By the end of this chapter, the reader will be able to:

1. Discuss the ways in which clinicians' values affect clinical encounters.
2. Describe the impact of system values, both institutional and community, on clinical encounters.
3. Discuss the ways in which client values affect clinical encounters.
4. Define cultural interpreter, translator, and group spokesperson, and identify the differences among these three types of culture brokers.
5. Discuss the potential values and drawbacks of using each type of culture broker.
6. Describe the ways in which clinicians serve as culture brokers.
7. Describe strategies for dealing with incomplete information in cultural encounters.
8. Describe methods for learning the client's perspective.

THE STORY OF LIA LEE

After Lia Lee returned home from foster care, the Lees were visited regularly by Jeanine Hilt, a social worker from child protective services. Jeanine was the only American in an official capacity who asked the Lees about their approaches to healing. She was also one of the few professionals who did not characterize the Lees as "close-mouthed and dim" (Fadiman, 1997, p. 112). The Lees reported that Jeanine was sympathetic and concerned. Jeanine took them on as a special challenge and tried to help them by working out a specific schedule that she posted on a wall. This was a good idea, though the Lees could not read it without the help of one of their children.

At age 4, about 6 months after returning home, Lia fell off a swing at her day care center and went into status epilepticus, an unremitting grand mal seizure of several hours' duration. When her blood level of medication was checked, it was clear that her parents were giving her the medication as prescribed. Lia aspirated fluid during this episode and, exposed to an opportunistic bacterium during hospitalization, developed an infection. When the infection resolved she was sent home, but 3 weeks later she was readmitted with a fever and another bout of seizures of longer duration. Staff members were convinced that the Depakene was not working, so other efforts were made to treat the seizures.

Two months later, Lia had a major seizure. The Lees brought Lia to the hospital in an ambulance, rather than employing their usual method of carrying her in their arms. They felt that the ambulance arrival would force the staff to take the problem more seriously. It took 20 minutes longer to get her there than when they carried her because the EMT, attempting to deal with a life-threatening situation, took an unusually long time to depart from the Lees' home to the hospital. No one took her temperature, and diarrhea and a low platelet count were noted without comment. Valium was administered in an attempt to bring the seizure under control. Despite the aggressive medical treatment, Lia seized for almost 2 hours (20 minutes is considered life-threatening).

Through the entire situation, Nao Kao expressed his view that it was the hospital that was making Lia sicker. He was convinced that they were providing the wrong treatment—a view that went unheard at the hospital.

Summarized from Fadiman, A. (1997). *The spirit catches you and you fall down.* New York: Noonday Press.

VALUES REVISITED

In an earlier chapter you learned that value orientations have a major role in forming our expectations about what experiences mean and in constructing evaluations of them. For example, you may be one of the many people with a values orientation toward communal helping. This orientation may make you more likely to volunteer at a local food bank or encourage you to participate in recycling programs. It might also mean that when you go to a party you expect to help the hosts clear away the dishes. When you throw your own parties, you might consider people who do not offer such help to be rude or think them unfriendly. In other words, your expectations of how you and others should behave and your sense of what those behaviors mean, as well as your evaluation of the behaviors themselves, are linked inextricably with your value orientation.

People sometimes experience a conflict in values when they operate within systems that include contradictory values or elements from multiple systems. Contradictions exist in almost all systems; for example, we teach children to share crayons and at the same time teach them not to share answers on a test. Sometimes the consequences of such value conflicts become most obvious when cultures come into contact and individuals must resolve the conflicts in order to sustain meaningful lives.

For example, many Japanese students study in the United States, fully intending to return home with their new expertise and take up their lives where they left off. However, in the process of attending college and living in the midst of American culture, they begin to acquire, almost without knowing it, new values concerning issues such as the role and status of women, use of leisure time, styles of speaking, and so on. It has been reported (French, 2000) that these new perspectives and practices can cause considerable difficulty for returnees to Japan. They may not be allowed to have too much contact with customers, or may be shunned by coworkers or advised not to show their expertise in English. They may feel isolated or angry. Many decide to leave Japan and attempt to return to the United States.

Health and health care are arenas in which, even within the "same" cultural group, values can come into conflict. Within a single group, individuals participate in different cultural networks and interact within institutional or organizational contexts that bring their own value orientations into the interaction. In any clinical setting, for example, there are at least three general sets of cultural backgrounds present: those of the clinician, those of the client, and those of the health care institution or system that defines the setting. In this chapter we will explore how these value systems come into contact and how cultural influences may add even more complexity to the situation.

We have discussed two useful concepts that can help us think about these contacts, interactions, and conflicts. One way to think about the various systems in contact is to keep in mind the idea of vantage. As described in Chapter 5, any participant in an interaction operates from a specific, individual, multilayered vantage. As you work through the examples in this chapter, keep asking yourself: What is the vantage of this participant or that? How do the vantages of the participants differ? Mutual cultural accommodation, also described in Chapter 5, may be helpful in managing cultural interactions. Because all participants are in interaction, success depends on accommodating the different vantages. As you read, ask yourself: What are the possibilities for accommodation here? If I were the clinician, what could I do realistically to encourage accommodating practice?

Clinician Values

Part of the socialization that any health care provider undergoes during the professional training process is socialization into the values of a specific profession. Each profession builds its own web of rituals, values, behavioral norms, aesthetic foundations, and social hierarchies—some of the cultural components that define any human group. As a person becomes a speech pathologist, a clinical psychologist, or a social worker, that person generally adopts much of the **normative behavior** and values associated with that profession. For example, some professions claim a higher place on the overall hier-

archy of health care. Some place heavier importance on improved client performance and others on client satisfaction. Some health professionals encourage behavioral changes in the management of chronic conditions, whereas others encourage medication. The socialization to a profession adds a layer to the culture emergent in the individual (Figure 6-1).

Mattingly (1998) notes that within medicine and therapy, values differ by area of specialization. "Rehabilitation medicine in general and occupational therapy in particular fit precariously in the medical mold, requiring so much more active and collaborative relationship between clinician and patient than is the norm in biomedicine" (p. 78). However, even practice in the same area of specialization does not ensure that professionals will hold exactly the same values.

6-1. Think about your own chosen professional area. What are the two or three key values that are important to your identification as a member of that profession? What values are critical to your success in the profession?

6-2. How are you expected to relate to a client? How does your profession define a successful intervention with a client?

6-3. What are the expectations about how professionals in your field relate to other professionals in contact with the same client?

6-4. Now compare your list with one made by another student or colleague from a different health profession. Are there differences in your key values or expectations?

6-5. Together, imagine a client who might require you to reconcile those differences. How are the differences complementary? How may they help the client? Are any in direct conflict? How might that conflict be manifested and then resolved?

In addition to professional values, of course, any clinician brings her or his own web of cultural influences into the setting with the client. It is simply impossible to eliminate all the expectations, values, and judgments that are part of our identities, so we must not expect to do so. However possible and desirable it is to adopt a professional demeanor that

Q

Figure 6-1. Health care organizations offer settings for professional socialization to the structures and behavioral norms of the organizational culture.

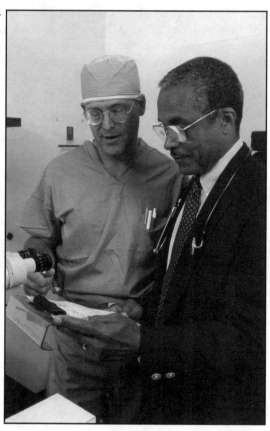

reduces the salience of our personal cultural influences, we cannot avoid at least some unconscious emotional responses that inevitably include evaluative judgments. These judgments can interfere with or even undermine our professional assessment. Part of adopting an ethnographic mindset in health care practice involves engaging in self-monitoring around the possibility of such cultural interference, especially when we are dealing with persons from unfamiliar backgrounds.

There is a difference between cognitive or professional or analytical understanding in a situation and emotional or subjective understanding. The goal of a professional must be to accept this difference and then manage it. Some beliefs and assumptions are so deeply embedded in our cultural experiences that they are tied to our physical response system. Recall the Hindu woman who ate a delicious casserole on her first trip to the United States and later vomited when she learned it was meat. This example is a fairly convincing demonstration of the connection between deeply ingrained values—eating meat is disgusting and wrong—and nearly uncontrollable physical reaction.

A cognitive understanding that meat is a valued protein source in some societies; that vegetari-

anism is a cultural choice with ethical, ritual, and religious components for some adherents; and that choosing to be an omnivore does not necessarily make a person evil may well allow an individual to exert control over the physical reaction. These understandings, along with motivations such as a desire to be polite or behave with a professional demeanor and persona, may even eliminate the physical revulsion altogether. Developing this capacity for self-control is one of the principal advantages of education about human difference and of ethnographic training. Such education can inculcate the valuable lesson that there is a difference in the sense of self and the expression of self.

6-6. Have you ever had the experience of having to control your own emotional reactions to something a person did or said? Reflect on that experience. What values were in conflict? What emotions were aroused? How did you control your emotional response? Why did you choose to do so?

6-7. If the person you were responding to was a client or a supervisor, how important were professional values in guiding your behavior?

Q

Q 6-8. Is there an important aspect of your sense of self that you conceal from coworkers? From clients? Reflect on why and how you conceal this aspect of self. What behavior do you avoid that might expose it? What values conflict is at the root of your choice to conceal?

Although each individual profession has its own constellation of assumptions and values, a critical element in socialization to almost all types of professional practice in the United States is the adopting of a biomedical model of physical and emotional illness and health. Few practitioners would deny that the American medical system is based on an accurate and realistic understanding of health and illness and the human body. In this biomedical model, disease always has a definable (usually organic) cause, medical treatment is always preferred to the lack of such treatment, and the patient is responsible for at least some elements of his or her own health. Practitioners who fail to socialize properly to such fundamental beliefs generally do not persist in a health care profession (if they enter it at all), and those who later come to doubt these beliefs may opt out or be forced out of their profession. Any psychologist who routinely diagnosed clients with demon possession and offered exorcism rituals for treatment would soon find herself out of reimbursements, out of her group practice, and potentially out of her profession altogether as a matter of ethics board review.

The American Psychiatric Association's 1994 edition of *The Diagnostic and Statistical Manual of Mental Disorders* (DSM-IV) makes clear what constitutes an acceptable diagnosis. Although it includes an appendix listing culturally bound conditions, these are not part of the accepted diagnostic structure for practitioners. In fact, it is not at all clear what a professional is to do with this list. Consider the DSM-IV entry for *hwa-byung* in the box below.

Q 6-9. Does *hwa-byung* sound like any condition with which you are familiar?

6-10. Have you ever experienced this cluster of symptoms or known someone who did? If so, what did you call the problem? What sort of help, if any, did you seek?

The assumptions that undergird the socialization, incorporation, and persistence of health professionals into the health care fields are strongly culturally influenced. However real and scientific we may agree that a particular microbe is, the assumptions that govern how we name, treat, and think about the disease it causes are part of our cultural history and experience. When scientists must decide whether to retain a small sample of the smallpox virus, and the arguments turn on such issues as its value for future scientific research or its potential for germ warfare by terrorists, we have left the realm of objective reality and entered the complex realm of culture. Any health practitioner, in all contexts, is operating from some vantage in this realm and may be interacting with clients who do not share those beliefs.

A profound example of the cultural underpinnings of health beliefs is seen in situations in which a patient is in a persistent coma. Most professionals believe that the longer a coma continues, the less likely it is that the individual will regain consciousness. Professionals point to a substantial body of research data, as well as their own experience, to support this belief. However, it is not unusual to find families who believe that if they spend enough time with the individual, talking to him or her, perhaps praying, the person will improve. Just like professionals, they have a body of literature to which to point—the reports in the press about individuals who after months or even years regain consciousness. In such cases, the professionals firmly believe that coma is caused by damage to brain neurons and that brain neurons cannot regenerate. Families may believe that faith and the expression of love are powerful sources of healing that can overcome serious injury.

Nevertheless, a therapeutic diagnosis based on the biomedical model will almost certainly be

---

AN EXAMPLE FROM THE DSM-IV APPENDIX

Hwa-byung is a Korean syndrome that translates into English as "anger syndrome." It is attributed to suppressed anger. Among its symptoms are insomnia, fatigue, panic, fear of imminent death, indigestion, anorexia, and a feeling of a mass in the epigastrium (APA, 1994).

accepted as "the" diagnosis, regardless of what client preferences or family opinion may be. Within the health care system of the United States, the practitioner's diagnosis usually wins out in any case of conflict. That outcome will not necessarily mean that such conflicts will therefore be minimized or will not matter. It may be that the conflicts will be magnified, precisely because of this lack of congruence.

Even within the same culture, the practitioner's assumptions of what is valuable for a client may clash with the client's assumptions and judgments. For example, an occupational therapist, driven by his professional focus on function and self-care, may insist that a client with severe hand weakness learn and practice self-dressing procedures. This occupational therapist may not even realize that the client prefers to use only pullover clothing or does not mind having a family member button her shirts, so that she can spend more time reading. If the occupational therapist's values create a vantage from which the occupational therapist cannot even ask about the client's preferences in this area or if he disregards them, inevitably, conflict will be the result. Because the therapist's diagnosis and intervention plan will "win," the client may come to be considered noncompliant. The therapist's winning has only made his task—and the client's—more difficult.

As noted in Chapter 4, one area in which there has been recent change affecting the acceptance of the biomedical model in health care in the United States is the entrance of holistic philosophies into health practice and the use of alternative medical practice among professional providers. We may wonder why holistic or alternative health care models have come into competition with the biomedical model in our national culture at this particular point in our history. A large number of factors probably come into play, including demographic changes, uneasiness with new biomedical technologies, dissatisfaction with the corporatization of the relationship between health care providers and their patients, economic considerations, and a widening attention to spiritual, environmental, and quality of life matters that is translating into a concern with tradition, native cultures, and natural remedies. The important point is that this larger social change, as it emerges through client demand, could alter professional training and thus professional values in profound ways. Certainly, health professionals will confront aspects of this changing context in individual client interactions that may challenge the system of biomedically based values that are intrinsic to much contemporary practice.

As one example, consider the emergence of client-centered care (Law, 1998). This term refers to a philosophy that considers the client or health care consumer an active participant in treatment planning and intervention. The idea that the client might bring important information to the encounter and might have specific ideas about the goals of care is relatively new; previously, the assumption was that the provider, especially the physician, was to "cure" the person. This revised orientation is certainly not the first change, nor will it be the last, in value systems affecting both clinician and client beliefs and expectations.

System Values

Organizations, too, exist within a web of assumptions, expectations, and evaluations that reflect the competing influences of their employees, employee groups, clients, managers, owners, regulators, and various related institutions. We may think of these complex, interacting influences as a type of organizational culture. Practitioners are always working within settings defined, supported, and constrained by such organizational cultures.

Consider the difference between **community hospitals** and **academic medical centers** (Osterweis, McLaughlin, Manasse, & Hopper, 1996). Community hospitals tend to be relatively small and located within the community they serve. They emphasize treatment of simple, common medical disorders such as appendicitis. They often do a great deal of community outreach, providing educational programming and screenings. They typically do not do medical research, nor do they have large numbers of health care students (e.g., medical students and residents or nursing students). Academic medical centers, on the other hand, tend to be large complexes of buildings located in city centers, drawing patients from all over their geographic area and sometimes from across the nation or around the globe. Their missions include research and teaching. Patients in the two types of hospitals may have dramatically different experiences, as the behavior of professionals in the different systems varies greatly. Similarly, social service agencies differ from hospitals and from each other depending on funding source, location, and other variables. Outpatient clinics differ from inpatient facilities, sheltered workshops from schools, and so on.

6-11. You have probably visited, worked, or done clinical training in a variety of organizational settings. Choose the two with which you are

Q

most familiar and describe the organizational structure, interactional style, and core values or mission of each one. What impact did those differences have on your experiences in each one?

Q 6-12. Compare your two settings with those of a colleague or classmate. What differences and similarities do you find in the structure, style, and values across the four settings? How are the differences and similarities related to the differences and similarities in experience that you and your colleague reported?

Sometimes traditional organizational cultures operate within a relatively unconsidered set of assumptions, which, when challenged, produce discomfort. For example, consider the case of a center that provides services to the blind and visually impaired that has employed mostly sighted staff; this history has produced the default assumption that "people who work here can see." Recently, more persons with impaired vision have begun to work in paid positions at the center. In the bustle of organizing tasks for a large children's party sponsored by the center, one sighted staffer asked one who was visually impaired, "Why don't you pour the punch?" The partially sighted person pointed out that in order to do so, he would have to put his finger in each cup to determine when it was full and that perhaps another task would suit him better. Unthinkingly, the sighted staffer suggested that the legally blind staffer take the party photographs instead. The sighted staffer's vantage was obviously founded on a very strong assumption about likely employees at the center. Upon reading such an example, we may be surprised at the insensitivity or inattention of the sighted staffer. However, what we should notice is the power of assumptions and the values they reflect, to control our perceptions. Values, as we have seen, are part of vantage and make some information invisible.

In many ways, and sometimes to a large extent, the values of practitioners have been closely aligned with the values incorporated in the organizations and institutions within which they work. One of the critical problems in health care in the United States today concerns the increasing gap between the values of health care providers themselves and the managers or corporations who now control much of the delivery of health care. Prioritization of financial outcomes for corporate stockholders has meant that practitioners experience lessened autonomy—

an extremely valued element for some professions—and may be subjected to greater restrictions or scrutiny. For example, care providers may be required to provide more justification for treatment plans or are allowed only a preset number of sessions with a client, regardless of the client's or the clinician's views on the matter. There may even be specified goals from which the clinician is to choose. The role of major insurance conglomerates and managed care organizations in setting fees, establishing preferred drug lists, and determining whether tests will be permitted is increasingly a matter of debate and one that has grown in acrimony. Changes in health care economics and advances in medical procedures are sources of conflict inside organizations and in public discourse. It is possible to view these conflicts as the results of real cultural contrasts—contrasts incorporated into interactions in which underlying assumptions and evaluations do not concur. Mattingly (1998) uses the term **underground practice** to describe how professionals can adhere to organizational dicta while finding ways to meet client needs that do not conform to those dicta.

As an example, consider the dilemma of a home health social worker whose intervention is constrained by very specific limitations on the set of intervention goals that are covered by Medicare. The social worker has undoubtedly been educated to address the well-being of the client in many spheres; Medicare, however, is prepared to pay only for those interventions that enable the individual to live at home. If the client is becoming depressed because of limited social interaction, the social worker may not be able to address this through community-based activities, but might instead address this concern in the context of an interview for which the main purpose is identification of sources of housekeeping help. Thus, although Medicare might not pay for interventions focused on social support, the social worker has employed "underground" techniques to ensure the client's well-being.

The notion of underground practice raises ethical dilemmas for clinicians, but the underlying message is one that practice has reflected for years. Effective clinicians know that they must address multiple health concerns in an efficient fashion. Time spent working on a nutritional plan, for example, can also be spent exploring issues of social support. The dietitian might inquire about who might share meals with the client, thus enhancing satisfaction with meal time and thereby increasing the likelihood that the client will maintain adequate nutrition.

Unfortunately, sometimes system values are in direct conflict with the values of service recipients. On occasion, these conflicts may result in the creation of new systems. In the 1970s, for example, therapists in rehabilitation settings were extremely focused on enabling newly disabled individuals to live independently in the community. Their definition of independence was that the individual could do all his or her own self-care. Many individuals with disabilities disputed this definition, asserting that they should be able to use personal assistants to provide their self-care so that they could conserve energy to accomplish other activities that they valued more. When they were unable to alter the beliefs of the therapists serving them, they established the Independent Living Movement (Seelman, 1999). The movement resulted in the creation of a new organizational entity, Services for Independent Living (SIL).

The system values of SIL were quite different from those of traditional rehabilitation centers, although in the intervening years the two have moved somewhat closer together. SIL has lobbied for readers for individuals with visual impairments and signers for individuals with hearing impairments. Rehabilitation services now also focus on such environmental modifications rather than adhering to their earlier insistence that the individual learn to function without such supports. Cultural difference may suggest alternative ways of structuring activities and environment. Compare Figures 6-2 and 6-3 and imagine how these might inform a practitioner concerned with material mobility issues.

In the past, changing organizational or system cultures was usually no easy or rapid task, but the recent history of American medical care has shown how changes in the various external impinging influences—emergence of health maintenance organizations, changes in Medicare reimbursement practice, legislative scrutiny, corporate mergers, and hospital closings—can occur relatively rapidly. Such changes themselves can alter system design and practice, but without altering the system's internal culture. The 1997 changes in Medicare billing guidelines reduced much physical therapy intervention by limiting reimbursement. The profession of physical therapy was immediately affected by these changes, which led to lay-offs and shrinking enrollments in training programs. As relationships among the parties in an organization shift as a result of these external changes, values come into conflict. For example, therapists were instructed by hospital financial offices about mechanisms for maximizing reimbursement through careful adherence to restrictive treatment schedules. For therapists educated to provide the needed service regardless of the time it takes, being told to restrict treatment to brief sessions was objectionable.

Another example is the change in the practice of psychiatry as psychotropic medications have become more readily available. Psychiatrists now find themselves spending most of their time prescribing medications rather than listening to their clients and working with them to address emotional concerns. Likewise, nurses now spend much more of their time supervising aides and assistants rather than providing direct care to clients. The change has left many nurses feeling uncomfortable about their ability to adequately care for patients they may have seen only briefly. The sense of being at odds with one's institutional culture can create conflicts for a practitioner and can affect decision-making around the client.

6-13. Can you think of recent news in your community or region that illustrates how health care institutions are changing (e.g., notices of hospital closings or medical center expansion)? What values—community, institutional, practitioner—does your example bring into conflict? How might a practitioner from your profession be affected by the changes? How can the practitioner understand the conflicts among values as cultural ones, in the sense we mean here?

6-14. Suppose that you are part of a large group practice under a for-profit, managed care structure. Imagine that a directive comes down from top management limiting all diagnostic testing for a condition treated in your practice to the three most common tests in the field. How might this directive come into conflict with your profession's values? What underground practices might result from that conflict?

It is sometimes easy to overlook the strength and persistence of system cultures and the sources of conflict they present in times of rapid social change. We see similar stresses in other major institutions in our society, as when mainstream religions grapple

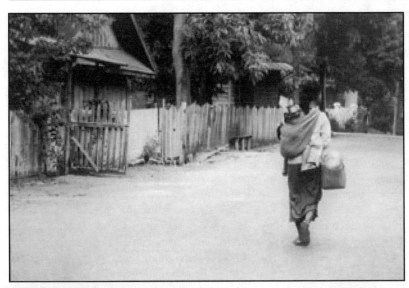

Figure 6-2. A mother carries a baby in Thailand. Photo courtesy of Wendy Schmidt.

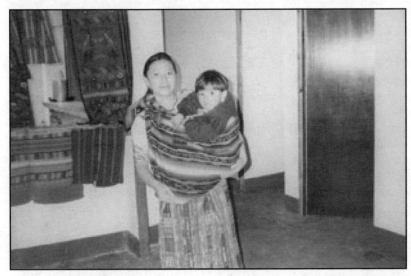

Figure 6-3. A Guatemalan Maya woman holds her child in a "carrying cloth."

with sexual orientation issues or universities cope with technological demands. The multicultural nature of American society predicts that among these institutions, there will always be smaller contending groups—more orthodox versus more liberal, for example—whose divergent views may further complicate the way system culture is perceived or evaluated.

The current controversy around autopsies is one example. There are some diseases, such as Alzheimer's, for which no diagnostic tests yet exist. The presence of the disease can only be confirmed by an examination of brain tissue. Researchers looking for information on the disease depend on autopsy results to provide it. Thus, every patient with suspected Alzheimer's is viewed as a potential research resource by the health field. Practitioners consider the autopsy essential to the progress of efforts to pre-

vent, treat, and diagnose the disease. Family members, on the other hand, may have different views. Religious groups such as Orthodox Jews or cultural groups like the Navajo oppose autopsy under any circumstances.

6-15. With a partner, role play the conversation between a bereaved family member of a patient with Alzheimer's disease and a health care worker seeking an autopsy that the family member opposes. Afterward, list the value claims made by each side. Identify each value used in the dispute as personal, professional, or institutional in basis.

Q

Conflicts in values cannot often be resolved simply by explaining their foundations because neither side can really accept the premises of the other.

In even more complex cases, an agent or group may propose to speak for all its members on such an issue, attempting to enforce dogmatic positions based on claims about group-wide values. Individual members of the group may hold divergent views. A health care professional may also be a group member yet have divergent opinions as compared with the group. When called upon to advise patients, certain situations may cause conflicts in values that can encompass the system, the practitioner, and the client.

In hospitals affiliated with a religious group that opposes abortion, for example, abortions may be prohibited. One nurse reported the dilemma she faced when a woman presented to the emergency room of the Catholic hospital at which she worked. The woman was diagnosed with an ectopic pregnancy. This type of pregnancy represents a life-threatening situation, but there is currently no way to save the embryo that has implanted inappropriately in the fallopian tube rather than the uterus. Catholicism is firmly opposed to abortion and perceives surgery for ectopic pregnancies as a form of abortion. Therefore, the woman had to be transferred to another hospital for the needed procedure, leaving the nurse concerned that during the transfer the medical emergency would become worse. Her personal values were in conflict with those of the organization.

Client Values

Clinicians are often caught between system cultures and professional cultures in conflict. Into this mix comes the client, who brings along his or her own culture emergent, a complex of cultural influences. To the extent that those cultural threads involve cultural backgrounds that are different from the care provider's experience, the interaction may take on cross-cultural overtones and involve unexpected or hidden conflicts. In any case, even when the client and the clinician share many characteristics, the roles of patient and health care provider are sufficiently different in and of themselves to produce the potential for misunderstanding, values conflict, and evaluations that are based on criteria relevant only to one or the other.

Patients are often in distress, in pain, and afraid, and always in a position subordinate both to the provider and to the system. From this perspective, patients and clinicians are almost invariably required to negotiate their interactions from an unequal footing. It is important for providers to keep this power differential in mind. Feelings of powerlessness, anger at being in a position of subordination, and reluctance to challenge the provider can have drastic consequences for patient care. Here is where the empathetic and nonjudgmental aspects of the ethnographic perspective can guide a clinician to imagine this unequal footing and act to counter it, exploring the client's assumptions, goals, and fears. Even without time to delve too deeply into details, the projection of empathy and honest curiosity may provide an opening for the client to be more direct or expressive.

The ethnographic mindset cannot easily coexist with the **depersonalization** that often accompanies practitioner training in some fields and the pressures of care settings in all fields. Attention to the "whole person humanity" of the client, the result of fully believing in the interconnectedness of all the elements of cultural, individual, and biological components, is the foundation upon which an ethnographic perspective is built. Through its insistence on self-checking, reflection, analysis, and comparison, the ethnographic mindset in itself provides a defense against the problems of over-attachment and emotional overload that are the dangers against which depersonalization is deployed.

Patients are also people in contexts of human relationships. That is, a care provider is almost never dealing just with the client. Almost certainly there will be other people involved in the person's care and decision-making processes. Family members, caretakers, close friends, even co-workers may become involved in discussions around the clinician's recommendations, treatments, and interactions. All of these individuals have their own vantages and, potentially, their own agendas, which may be in conflict with those of the clinician, the health care system, and the client. Such a situation may manifest itself in conflicts over compliance or treatment decisions, for example, and considerable pressure may be brought to bear on the client and on the provider to align with one or another of these conflicting agendas.

One therapist in a school system worked primarily with students who had identified learning disabilities. She developed a carefully constructed home program to be implemented by parents. The program included a series of exercises to be provided by parents, specific kinds of sensory stimulation, and a list of "effective" parenting strategies. What she failed to take into account was that she was giving her instructions to parents in a community comprised mostly of two-career families and single-parent families. Neither group had time for her 2- to 3-hour home program.

Q 6-16. Imagine that you are the care provider in this (or a similar) situation. What might you need to do to develop an effective and appropriate alternative intervention? Consider what information you would need and how to get it. What compromises might you have to make between your professional ideals and this reality? What kinds of assumptions might you have to change (e.g., about the parents, the structure of the intervention, or the schedule) in order to implement the new intervention successfully?

Similar conflicts may arise in the case of an elderly patient with a terminal condition whose children and grandchildren may encourage all possible treatments, even the most experimental or unlikely to succeed. Although the patient may not truly want these procedures, pressure to undergo them may be applied by his or her children and grandchildren. The children and grandchildren, in their own distress and grief, may see applying pressure as the right thing to do to preserve the values of the family or of the religious or ethnic group with which they identify. A provider may feel only an obligation to the individual client but must never forget that the client is receiving other information and being given other options from a multitude of surrounding sources. To the extent that some of the sources are closed to the clinician's understanding because of cultural difference, the clinician will have difficulty in negotiating the appropriate option with the client. Sometimes, although it can create even greater difficulty by posing ethical dilemmas within the provider's world view, the clinician may be called upon to adjudicate such situations.

An example of such a situation was reported by a nurse of our acquaintance. She described the case of a 93-year-old woman brought to the hospital for amputation of a gangrenous leg, the result of chronic diabetes of many years' duration. This was to be the woman's second lower-extremity amputation. The surgeon had made it clear to the woman and her two daughters that without the surgery the woman would die in the near future. The daughters were adamant about the importance of surgery; the woman said very little on admission. Several hours later, however, she called the nurse and tearfully told her that she did not want the procedure. She said, "I've lived a good life. I'm ready to go. I know what this surgery is like and I can't face it." She begged the nurse to intercede with the surgeon, whose professional culture dictated that surgery should be done whenever the immediate condition could be resolved in this way and with her daughters, who had been raised in a religious environment in which any form of euthanasia was considered a sin. In this role, the nurse is asked to become what ethnographers would call a cultural broker.

BROKERING INTERACTIONS

A **cultural broker** is a person who serves go-between functions at the edges of cultural groups in contact. Ethnographers of traditional communities have described many types of broker functions and the types of individuals who perform them. Traders, for example, are often cultural brokers. Their role in transferring goods between two dissimilar groups offers them opportunities to introduce new ideas, material objects, and customs into the cultural mix. They often interpret the behavior of members of each group to the other. Because they are usually native to one group but have some sort of language skill with the other, even if it is only a partial knowledge or trading language, they have specialized expertise that is not shared with other members of either group. Such individuals are invaluable in situations of culture contact. They are also often marginalized within the native culture and behave in ways that do not always conform to traditional expectations. They also may be marginalized in the dominant or colonial culture.

6-17. Think about how a person gets to be a cultural broker. What attributes and experiences might fit a person for such a role? Why is it likely that a cultural broker would be marginalized in both the native and non-native cultures? **Q**

6-18. Whom do you know who might be called a cultural broker? Have you ever found yourself in such a role?

Curiosity, tolerance, professional need, a certain degree of willingness to entertain ambiguity and incomplete information, and the experience to recognize and interpret pattern may all be part of the mix of attributes that characterize potential cultural brokers, just as they are for ethnographers and people who think like them. These attributes and experiences may make an individual more suited to cross-cultural interaction, but they may also cause the person to behave in ways that are not customary within the native group. This slight marginalization is precisely what fits the broker for the role. It may also make the individual and others uncomfortable with it.

Types of Brokers

Cultural Interpreters

A type of broker who may be found in health care settings is the **cultural interpreter**, usually a person who is a member of the same group as the client but who is somewhat familiar with health care procedures, systems, and values in the dominant society. This person, too, is inevitably someone with his or her own unique experiences with each group and who may have adapted his or her behaviors, values, and beliefs in the process of acquiring those experiences. Although perhaps often perceived by others as a neutral or objective participant, such an individual in fact has a particular vantage, with all the elements that implies, and is no more neutral than any of the other participants.

Translators

Another frequent specialist who may be brought into health care settings to broker an interaction is a **foreign language translator**. Here again, not only is there the potential for conflicting agendas or values, but there is the additional issue of skill level. Just because a patient speaks Spanish does not necessarily mean that anyone who speaks Spanish and English can translate the patient's language. Many languages, Spanish among them, have great internal variation in pronunciation, vocabulary, and meaning. These variations have the potential to disrupt rather than to improve communication. Moreover, sharing a language does not address the issue of other cultural factors. The case of the Indiantown Maya found on page 119 offers a particularly poignant case in point.

Recall Lia Lee. As her contact with the medical system unfolded, a number of foreign language translators (e.g., a cousin of the Lees, a staff member in the hospital) were employed, as were two different cultural brokers. The language translators differed in their understanding of English and Hmong, and the cousin had no more understanding of medical jargon than did the Lees. As the older Lee children learned English, their parents began to use them as language translators as well.

The first cultural broker who worked with the Lees was a second-generation Hmong woman who was married to a wealthy man. Although prominent in Merced, the woman was mistrusted in the Hmong community because of her degree of acculturation. Thus, although hospital staff assumed she could assist, what they did not perceive was that she had negative views about some of the Lees' behaviors. She conveyed her disapproval to them in many of her interactions.

The more successful broker was a cultural interpreter who worked with Fadiman (1997) as she gathered data for her book on the case. Also a second-generation Hmong, this woman had cultivated positive relations in the Hmong community and maintained her ties to Hmong tradition. She also recognized the limits of her knowledge of medical jargon and procedures, and tried to inform herself about them. Perhaps most important, she was aware that the Lees' experience was not identical to her own, and she was able to suspend judgment.

Even in situations where both parties speak the same language and come from similar cultural backgrounds, translation may be needed. The professional jargon of health professionals can also be opaque even to a client who is speaking the same basic language. Sometimes attempts to remedy the distancing effects of jargon or to correct for possible misinterpretation do not work out the way they are intended. We know of an elderly Romanian woman with a slow-growing terminal colon tumor who was being pressed by family members to consider a surgical procedure that would have possibly added a year or two to the 2-year prognosis she had received. At 91 years of age, she also had to reckon with the 50% chance that the surgery itself would kill her. In the discussion of the procedure and its outcome, the phrase "and you'll have to wear a bag" was used to describe the resulting colostomy. The woman nodded at this statement and raised no questions.

Later, in a discussion with her daughter, it was discovered that she had no idea to what the phrase referred. A modest and laconic woman, she had never discussed such matters with anyone before, and whatever image was created by the phrase "a bag," it was not a colostomy bag. When she heard it fully described, she was appalled and felt it was a strong deterrent to the surgery. Without this unplanned conversation, it is possible that this patient might have undergone the surgery and awakened to an unexpected reality.

The health care provider and the woman's relatives no doubt believed that by using an informal lay phrase they were communicating clearly to the client, fully informing her of the consequences of the choice of surgery. In fact, they had overestimat-

THE INDIANTOWN MAYA

Indiantown is a community in South Florida that has traditionally served as a labor transport point, originally for Native Americans (hence the town's name) and, more recently, for Caribbean migrants. Its small resident population (about 1,800 in 1980) includes whites and blacks. In the mid-1980s, a local church began to sponsor Mayan refugees fleeing the violence of the Guatemalan civil war. Suddenly the population doubled, and the new arrivals included many elderly people, women, and small children, who quickly became clients at the various local social service agencies, health clinics, and nearby hospitals.

Because they were primarily identified as "Guatemalans" (rather than as Mayans), they were assumed to be Spanish speakers. Many, especially the men, did know some Spanish, but most were monolingual in a Mayan language and spoke only rustic varieties of Spanish. The call for translators produced a new job opportunity for Spanish-speaking bilinguals in South Florida, most of whom are Cuban or Puerto Rican. The Caribbean varieties of Spanish—spoken rapidly with dropping of specific consonants, different patterns of vowel reduction, and regionally distinct vocabulary and slang—are quite different from those of Guatemalan Spanish. Their Caribbean and South Florida cultural backgrounds were very different as well, as were the attitudes of these sophisticated urbanites toward the "rustics" with whom they were now dealing. In any case, when clients turned out not to speak Spanish after all, everyone was at a loss in managing the encounter. There have been many accounts of the difficulties this mismatch produced. The availability of translators for the Mayan language that the newcomers actually spoke was almost nil.

As in many immigrant communities, the Indiantown Maya soon found that their children were rapidly learning English. By speaking the Mayan language at home and English outside, the children were skipping the acquisition of Spanish altogether. The children then came to be the translators for their older monolingual family members in various settings. Now, for purposes of health care, modest Mayan women might find themselves disrobed in front of their preteen children, who translated intimate details to strangers. Besides the natural discomfort with the health care setting and the providers, these patients suffered the additional indignity of revealing to their children aspects of their lives that no Mayan woman would normally discuss with a child. The effects of these experiences on the families were significant. The child's new role altered the balance of power and traditional roles within the family's organization, disorienting the parents and creating unaccustomed problems with discipline, privacy, and familial obligations. Thus, the circles of consequence spread from the health care arena into other spheres of life and eventually came back to the health provider in the form of "noncompliant" patients who refused treatment.

Adapted from Burns, A. F. (1993). *Maya in exile: Guatemalans in Florida*. Philadelphia: Temple University Press.

---

ed her experience of the world of colon disease, partly by not taking into account the cultural patterns associated with some Romanian women's way of talking about personal body matters and partly by assuming that a common euphemism would be widely understood. This example helps underscore the value of questioning every assumption and of cross-checking the data on the patient's understanding and interpretation of the provider's talk. Even where there is little apparent cultural difference, the differences of experience and expectation can be vast.

Q

6-19. What might you advise the provider in this example to do differently? Can you think of a similar example from your own experience or practice?

Such communication problems can work in both directions. Consider, for example, the case of a physician assistant from Indianapolis who had just started work in a community clinic in rural West Virginia. An 82-year-old-man was brought into the clinic by his four daughters, who said he was feeling bad and was "running off" several times a day. The physician assistant's first thought was that the man was experiencing the kind of wandering that is common in individuals who are developing dementia. It took close questioning to learn that in Appalachian English "running off" refers to having diarrhea. If the physician assistant had not been attentive to the possibility of misunderstanding, he might have failed to address the client's needs.

It is always easy to make assumptions about understanding. One school system psychologist, knowing that she was working with a parent who was also a psychologist, explained the child's learning deficit in terms of "disparate scores on the WISC" and other technical jargon. She was unaware that the mother, a practitioner with the elderly, not with children, felt uncomfortable with the jargon used in pediatric circles.

Group Spokespersons

In addition to cultural interpreters and translators, a third type of person can intervene to try to broker a health care interaction, perhaps without being physically present. This person is the individual (or sometimes an organization) who claims the role of **spokesperson** for a group of which the patient is an assumed member. Religious authorities, tribal elders, and public figures associated with a recognized organization can all emerge in the role of representing a member of an ethnic or social group, usually by making pronouncements on the ethical dimensions of an issue. These figures gain credibility outside the group and may be relied on for guidance by institutions, ethicists, and individuals. However, there are important questions about the ways in which individual and cultural values intersect in these cases. The most significant ones concern the problems of defining membership in the relevant group and adjudicating the contested identities and values that may come into play (Davis, 2000).

Consider the case of a newly graduated bioethicist from the Midwestern United States without much experience with Judaism who took a position with an institution in New York City, where her likely client base was largely Jewish. To prepare herself culturally, she read some of the extensive literature on bioethical concerns reflecting a Jewish perspective. Almost all of this literature is written by members of the Orthodox branches of Judaism, whose positions on many issues, such as autopsy, abortion, and genetic testing, are conservative. Unfortunately for the bioethicist, her clientele mostly consisted of Jews from the Reform branches, whose views are decidedly more mixed, more liberal, and held with just as much conviction. Her incorrect assumption had been that Jewish authorities spoke for Jews. She was not aware that there are many types of Jewish authorities, whose authority is relevant only for some of the many Jewish groups. She also failed to realize that her individual clients might represent a wide array of Jewish identities with their associated systems of values and beliefs (Davis, 1994).

Some Native American spokespersons have opposed the participation of tribal members in genetic research. Because many Native American groups have legally constituted tribal governments, it has been relatively simple for researchers to adopt the notion of "culturally appropriate authorities" as consultative bodies whose permission may or must be sought for the conduct of research. Not all Native Americans belong to or participate actively in such tribal affiliations, however, and not all individuals share the ideals or values of the governmental spokespersons.

6-20. Reflect on your own views applied to situations like this one. What rights do individuals who may be construed as group members have to agree to procedures or research protocols that group spokespersons oppose? What obligation do therapists or researchers have to inform individuals of the views of the "group" to which they might appear to be related as part of the discussion of consent? What do you think is the proper role of a health provider in assisting individual clients with these culturally influenced dilemmas?

6-21. Imagine you are working with parents who have learned through amniocentesis that the child they are expecting may have Down syndrome. Their options are to continue the pregnancy or to abort the fetus. What arguments might be mounted by the parents and their families, neighbors, and spiritual advisors either to abort or to continue the pregnancy? What value systems and what specific values may come into conflict during the decision-making process? Can you find a justification for each point of view?

6-22. How do you view the various arguments you developed for this case from the perspective of your own values as a practitioner? As a parent?

6-23. What is your profession's position on the question of whether you may advise the parents on the issue? Do you think that different cultural groups might have different views of this situation?

Figure 6-4. Professionals often find themselves brokering interactions among family members during family conferences like this one.

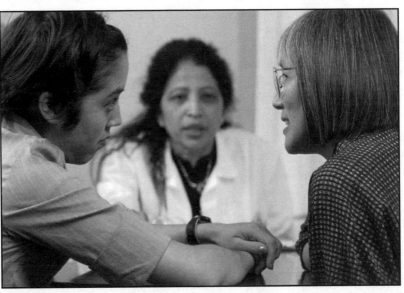

The Clinician as Broker Between the Client and the System

Although there are situations in which a designated culture broker (e.g., a family or community member) is brought into a health care situation, most often health care providers themselves serve as brokers between the client and the system. The medical system in the United States is profoundly frightening and unfamiliar to many citizens, even those who are not juggling additional factors such as extreme linguistic or cultural difference. In our view, it is the provider's obligation to assist clients in understanding aspects of the system, including its cultural norms, values, and expectations, that impinge on a client's ability to make well-informed decisions, manage their own health situation, and maneuver within the different arenas of the hospital, clinic, or practice group (Figure 6-4).

No professional standard of ethics requires professionals to intervene in clients' personal situations or to pressure them toward a particular decision or to find alternative methods to remedy system-created dilemmas. However, all such standards explicitly require that professionals offer the best care possible. This requirement demands that a practitioner recognize the conflicts in cultures and values that inevitably occur among the client, the system, and the profession, and make every effort to take them into account when determining care. We have more to say about the pragmatic implications of this stance in the next chapter, but it is useful to understand the role of broker as a necessary aspect of professional identity for all health care professionals.

Regardless of your own professional positioning and personal preferences, clients in distress and under pressure may request your assistance or advice when making difficult decisions. In these situations it is even more crucial to adopt the ethnographic perspective to help you manage yourself and the situation. Asking questions to gather pertinent information, suspending judgment while you try to see how the other person's perspective makes sense within a coherent system of values and beliefs, being alert to the role of cultural factors in the process, and being aware of your own vantage are all strategies to make you maximally helpful and minimally biased as you interact with persons in a less powerful position who are under stress and pressure dealing with difficult and complex matters. A significant component of thinking in this way is to learn to envision alternative explanations for sets of behaviors. This capacity for surprise—the ability to notice and accept that your own interpretation is not the only one available—is an important attribute for a culturally adept practitioner. Thinking about alternatives in interpretation and in intervention is a good way to practice the ethnographic mindset and also to learn more about the ways different groups of people understand the same sets of behaviors.

ENVISIONING ALTERNATIVES IN EXPLANATIONS AND INTERVENTIONS

The United States medical system already incorporates the concept of alternative explanation for disability or disease within its own structures and categories. To see how this variation is manifested, think about the varied interpretations of low back pain given by various practitioners. If you take your aching back to a chiropractor, the reason for your pain may be explained in terms of your body being out of alignment. The office may have skeletal charts on display, and the treatments will be described as methods of realigning vertebral and other major skeletal systems. The practitioner will take responsibility for accomplishing this alignment, and advice for home care may involve little more than suggestions for postural changes.

In a physical therapist's office, however, you might be told that your back aches because you have weak muscles or a disc problem. If the problem is chronic, you may be shown a diagram of the musculature of the lower spine. Your treatment will involve a program of exercises designed to strengthen the involved muscles, and the responsibility for improvement will largely be yours, governed by how well and regularly you perform the assigned practice.

If you then take your same pain and body to an acupuncturist, you may be diagnosed as suffering the consequences of a blockage in the flow of *qi* (sometimes spelled *chi*), a system of energy flow that is fundamental in Chinese medicine, within which acupuncture is a common modality of treatment. You may see large charts of the human body with energy lines and pressure points illustrated, perhaps with labels in languages other than English. The practitioner will treat you by assisting in the unblocking of *qi*, using tiny needles inserted into your body at predetermined points, which may not even be near the area of the pain. Your role and responsibility for healing may be in the form of mental exercises, such as meditation, or in the form of rearrangement of your work or living space.

Each of these three professional fields—chiropractic, physical therapy, and acupuncture—has a coherent understanding of the body, a tradition of training and practice, a body of supporting literature and research, and a well-integrated system of diagnosis and treatment. Other practitioners who treat chronic back pain also exist, of course, including surgeons, psychologists, and massage therapists.

Q 6-24. Think for a moment about the example. Can you define a set of underlying assumptions that might govern each of the professions mentioned? How are the assumptions in contrast?

6-25. If you were suffering lower back pain, which of the practitioner types might you be most likely to consult? What values or beliefs would govern your decision? Would you be willing to consult the others?

6-26. Do you know anyone who has consulted one of the other types of practitioners? Why might that person have made a decision different from your own? What kind of evidence of efficacy or what kind of situation might make you reconsider visiting a type of practitioner you have never previously consulted?

Research has suggested that each of these types of therapies may improve a case of lower back pain to about the same degree (Pittler, 1999). The outcomes seem largely dependent on such factors as the client's level of trust or acceptance of diagnosis and on the degree to which the pain itself is not associated with some other factor altogether (e.g., a psychosocial dysfunction such as depression).

6-27. For the types of practitioners not considered **Q** in detail—surgeons, psychologists, and massage therapists—can you develop a list of characteristics regarding probable diagnosis, treatment, and locus of control for improvement?

From this example, we can see that alternative interpretations of the origin of illness and alternative interventions designed to heal or relieve it exist. Such variations may not be particularly related to overt cultural factors. In fact, many health plans include acupuncture within the structure of covered providers, and many practicing acupuncturists today do not subscribe to the entire system of traditional Chinese philosophy concerning *qi*.

Differences in interpretation, and their influences, are not limited strictly to the practitioner's office. Consider the case of "The Man on the Street" that appears in the box on page 123.

Examples involving the contrasts created by individual, cultural, and social interpretations of health, wellness, disability, causation, diagnosis, treatment, and cure abound. Sometimes additional factors, including historical, political, and demographic ones, also play a role in constructing alternative explanations that can have an impact on health care. One of the most interesting current areas where we can see such a shift in explanation concerns menopause. On the whole, until the early 1900s, most women did not live to experience menopause. Poor nutrition, lack of proper sanita-

The Man on the Street

Imagine this scenario, based on an incident described to one of us by a psychologist friend. The scene is a downtown neighborhood in a northern city, in early evening. An elderly man, wearing a frayed black suit and white shirt, walks slowly along the sidewalk and then up the steps and onto a townhouse porch occupied by its two residents. The man gesticulates in unusual ways and makes unintelligible sounds. He does not respond to questions or to the residents' instructions to leave. The police are called.

- How many possible explanations can you think of for the man's behavior? If you were a police officer called in for a possible case of trespass, what questions might you ask and what sorts of observations might you make to determine whether the man's behavior is criminal?

Suppose that the police officer receives no answers to his questions. The townhouse owners become frightened and insist that something be done to remove the individual from their premises. The man is becoming increasingly agitated and loud.

- Imagine that you are the owner. What interpretation would you be most likely to make about the man's behavior? Imagine that you are the police officer. What interpretation would be the most likely one for you to make about the nature of the man's disturbance? What intervention would you probably choose to implement?

In this case, the man was considered to be behaving "bizarrely," and he was taken by the police to the forensics unit. There he was assessed as psychotic, and a decision was made to admit him to the emergency department of a psychiatric hospital for further evaluation.

- Reconsider the possible explanations you developed earlier. Was this explanation one that occurred to you? Can you now think of alternative explanations for the man's behavior?

At the hospital, an emergency room nurse overheard the man talking in an agitated and disjointed way to the intake personnel. She approached the police officers, the intake person, and the elderly man and said something to him that no one else heard. He immediately became calm, spoke to her, and she seemed to understand him. Imagine that you are the accompanying police officer.

- What new interpretations about the situation might now occur to you upon seeing this interaction?

The emergency room nurse was of Greek background and recognized the man's words as Greek, although somewhat distorted and ill-pronounced. It was later learned that the elderly gentleman was a recently arrived Greek immigrant who understood very little English. He was also hearing impaired, making it difficult for him to pronounce with complete intelligibility what little English he knew. His gestures were signed Greek. He had become lost while traveling to an appointment about a job. When he came onto the townhouse porch, he was asking to use the phone to call a taxi.

- Was any of this reality—his non-native cultural background, language, disability, purpose—part of your previously imagined interpretations? If not, what assumptions of yours do you think prevented you from imagining such an explanation for his behavior?
- What might have been the outcome for the elderly Greek man if the Greek-speaking nurse had not been on duty that night?

tion, unhygienic birthing circumstances, and prolific infectious disease all contributed to a low life expectancy. After World War II, due in large part to improvements in antibiotics, sanitation, and the distribution of medical care, life expectancy increased dramatically for both men and women, permitting a large number of women to live past the age of menopause.

Furthermore, at the same time, the Baby Boom (individuals born between 1946 and 1964) created an enormous cohort of females who would experience the full impact of these improvements. Many of these Boomer women also experienced the political and social changes spurred by feminism, which included various health-related movements toward greater participation in health decisions, greater awareness of women's health issues, and greater support for women's health research.

Outside the women's movement, other social pressures also affected perceptions of older women and of their expectations about aging and health. These included the trend toward earlier and more active retirements, the conflicts over unnecessary hysterectomies, and childbearing at a later age. The growth of the self-help movement provided sources and resources for alternate interpretations and interventions related to the symptoms and experience of menopause. Hormone replacement therapy became widely available, but conflicting research findings about its impact on other diseases, such as heart disease and breast cancer, made its reception less than unequivocally positive. Information about the roles given to post-childbearing women in other cultures and about the experiences of such women at menopause also became widespread.

It is thus no accident that in the 1990s, when the first Boomer women reached perimenopause, various reinterpretations of menopause began to emerge. A whole new range of medicines, supplements, devices, books, workshops, and programs that cater to the menopausal woman became available. Public discourse now accepts references to the process and its symptoms in everything from television advertising to stand-up comedy to newspaper cartoons to political campaigns. Research into menopause cross-culturally, as well as into the nuances of the precise physiologic course of bodily changes has expanded. Much more variety exists among the possible interpretations that an individual woman and her health care providers can make of her experience and expectations.

Any individual woman will make choices among these interpretations based on her personal and cultural values, personality, lifestyle, and the influences of other valued sources. Some women begin hormone replacement therapy early in perimenopause and continue to menstruate into their 70s, in some ways avoiding natural menopause altogether. Others adopt what they consider the "more natural" methods of herbal medicine to deal with menopausal symptoms. Still others denounce the medical model underlying notions of "loss" or "deficiency," look to the post-reproductive period as a time of personal growth and begin to explore new careers, activities, and forms of spirituality. Some women have even adapted the ceremonial rituals used by certain Native American groups to celebrate a woman's cessation of menstruation and her entry into the ranks of the valued elders. As the Boomer generation proceeds through this life phase, we may expect to see even more variability developing and even more potential for competition among ways of adapting to the process of menopause. This example suggests something of the complexity of the factors that interact in the process of value formation, value conflict, and value change.

These few examples have illustrated some aspects of the notion of alternative explanation or alternative interpretation. It is useful to assume that whatever interpretation you imagine correct can be challenged under the same facts, by an alternative set of assumptions, values, or experiences. When different cultural backgrounds are represented among the participants, it is essential to assume that your interpretation is not completely shared by at least some of the others. It is equally essential to assume that negotiating among these various interpretations to find the right intervention for the client is part of your brokering role. The client cannot usually do it and certainly cannot do it alone. Consider the case of "The Occupational Therapist and the Elderly Man" discussed in the box on page 125. As you cultivate the capacity for surprise and practice the questioning, hypothesizing, and checking skills of the ethnographic mindset, you will become more adept at identifying conflicts in interpretation and quicker at resolving them, even when, as is always the case, you do not have time to gather all the information you need.

DEALING WITH INCOMPLETE INFORMATION

Clinicians are always working in the absence of complete information when they work in culturally rich settings. There are few comparative data at hand on the issues raised in this book, because this area is a relatively new one, in which little research has been done within the contexts of professional practice. More importantly, information about others is never complete. Certainly, no health care provider, no matter how careful or detailed, no matter how sensitive or thorough, no matter how conscientious or inquisitive, can ever ask all the possibly relevant questions or even all the most relevant questions. You cannot always know which questions to ask, or you cannot ask enough questions, or you do not ask the right questions at the right time. You cannot alter any of these factors. It is simply not possible to ask all the relevant questions. Even professional ethnographers are not immune to this limitation. No ethnographer ever has full access to all the possible information about a community of

THE OCCUPATIONAL THERAPIST AND THE ELDERLY MAN

We know an occupational therapist (OT) who, during her first internship experience, was working with an elderly African-American man with diabetes whose leg had been amputated from just above the knee. The assumptions conveyed during the OT's training were that any amputee who could use a prosthesis would want to (or "should"), so she devoted herself to helping him learn how to wrap the stump so that it would fit into a prosthesis when the time came. This procedure was standard at the time the therapist was training a number of years ago. The man had also suffered a mild stroke and had some paralysis on one side, making the process of wrapping a difficult and slow one to master as well as to perform. The man was mild-mannered and kind, and the young OT was dedicated and persistent. Fortunately for her, however, the old man finally got the courage to reveal that he thought mobility with a wheelchair was sufficient for his lifestyle and that he never intended to get a prosthesis at all.

It had never occurred to the OT-in-training that his goals and intentions had been so different from the ones she assumed he had. Also fortunately for her, when she approached her supervisor for assistance on the matter of convincing her patient that a prosthesis would be better for him, the supervisor helped her see that the choices were the client's and that the valued activities in his life should dictate his decision. The supervisor also communicated the view that it was appropriate for an OT provider to help a client achieve his own goals, even if they were different from those anticipated or assumed by the profession's value system.

From that point on, this OT began to be interested in the issues surrounding the meanings of activities in individual lives and in the development of best-practice training methods that would help practitioners internalize an approach that emphasized the client-centered perspective. To this day, she values that early experience with a patient who was patient with her, but who impressed on her that she had not asked him the right questions.

study, because not even its own participants have such access to a culture's variety. Everyone, everywhere, is limited in cultural access by age, gender, status, occupational class, wealth, and many other factors.

One consequence of this inevitably limited database is that you cannot dwell on the lack of complete information. You must act, make decisions, make recommendations, treat, and help heal. One of the paradoxes of the ethnographic mindset relates specifically to finding ways to deal with the fact that information is limited, variable, contradictory, and dynamic. Adopting this perspective makes you uncomfortably aware of your own limitations of knowledge. However, it should also help you feel that you are increasingly equipped, through every interaction, to gather ever more information and to understand it ever more clearly. You will know you have achieved the perspective we are describing when you leave every interaction with more questions. Sometimes the empathetic and inquiring persona that you project as a consequence of adopting

this perspective will provide intangible help to the client, even when you make no changes in your treatment plan.

A good way to practice this perspective is to risk taking the client's vantage. Perhaps while you write up notes, think about, or discuss a difficult case, you can spend a few minutes imagining yourself in the position of the client. Try to imagine what questions you would have, what aspects of the therapeutic setting or interaction might have been confusing or frightening, and what fears you might have felt. Revisit your own questioning and conversation, imagining ways your behavior might have been received by a client who does not share your experience, training, or culture. Envision alternatives in your own behavior that might have improved communication or understanding. These moments of reflexive thinking, of self-reflection and analysis, and of putting yourself in the other person's place can help you develop the skills of creating alternative interpretations or using alternative strategies in your own behavior while you are working with a client. This mental work is also crucial to the process of assessment and evaluation that we discuss in Chapter 8. Begin now to practice it.

VALUES IN INTERACTION

In every interaction with other people, our value systems and theirs come into contact and possible conflict. With people very much like ourselves the potential for conflict may be slight, and, in general, these interactions confirm and strengthen our culturally grounded belief systems. Still, it is in these interactions that slight changes and reassessments may occur, contributing to the ongoing process of culture change. It is for this reason that we have said that culture is dynamic, or changing, and emergent, that is, constantly negotiated and constructed through individual interactions. When people are less like us, the potential for conflict between values grows, as does the potential for the assumptions that underlie them to be in conflict. We have suggested that taking a client's perspective, attending to the brokering dimensions of the therapist's role, and developing the skills required to envision alternative scenarios are all valuable ways to reduce such conflict and enhance the potential for compromise and accommodation. Sometimes an experience may occur early in a practitioner's work life that illustrates the importance of these capacities. Such an experience may transform a provider's understanding of his or her role in health care, as was the case for a young occupational therapist and her elderly client described in the box on page 125.

It is important to remember that not all interaction involving people from obviously different cultures necessarily involves cultural factors. Recently, one of us had the following experience while standing in line in an airport ladies' room. A middle-aged woman, wearing a sari and with the physical features of an East Indian, was standing by a sink, obviously trying to wash her hands. The sink was one of the new high-tech versions with only a faucet and no handles. The woman pushed perplexedly at the soap button and the faucet and the little metal circles on the side of the sink. She looked across the room and saw a person miming the act of putting hands directly under a faucet. She followed this hint and water came out. She washed

her hands and nodded her thanks as she left the room. This interaction, in spite of the obvious cultural and linguistic differences between the two participants, did not have any cultural identity components at work. It was based entirely on familiarity or lack of familiarity with a particular kind of plumbing technology, a familiarity not necessarily linked to any cultural attribute. The use of gesture to communicate owed more to the distance across the room than to linguistic differences. In fact, many of us can recall episodes in which we ourselves have been in precisely the same situation and received the same sort of help from a person who may have looked a lot like us.

This moment was a simple human interaction, one based on mutual sociability and a willingness to interact in the best available modality. Fortunately for ethnographers, travelers, and health care providers, most human interaction is characterized by these features, no matter what else may be going on. We can often depend on just that mutual humanity as the footing on which we can stand while we work through our differences. Such human interactions, based on mutual sociability, and on suspension of stereotypes and preconceived ideas, are also the kinds of interactions most likely to yield effective results in clinical settings.

6-28. Think about recent experiences you may have had in unfamiliar environments. What behaviors did you witness that puzzled you? As you reflect now on those puzzling experiences, try to remember how you found out what the behaviors meant. Did you ask someone? Observe and try to guess? Wait until someone told you?

6-29. Which of those experiences do you think were related to cultural difference or cultural misunderstanding? Which of them do you think were the result of simple lack of information and were not cultural in origin?

We now turn our attention to the enactment of these strategies in clinical practice. As you move to the next chapter, remember the importance of the ethnographic mindset and of active curiosity about your clients and yourself.

✎ Notes ✎

✎ NOTES ✎

Evaluating Clients and Designing Interventions in a Diverse World

CHAPTER OBJECTIVES

By the end of this chapter, the reader will be able to:

1. Identify culturally relevant factors important to assess during the evaluation process.
2. Discuss the advantages and disadvantages of using standardized instruments.
3. Describe ethnographic interviewing and the advantages and disadvantages of this method.
4. Describe methods for incorporating cultural information while setting intervention goals.
5. Discuss mechanisms for incorporating culture into intervention, including procedures for choosing and modifying activities or medical procedures.
6. Describe methods for negotiating with clients around intervention and for ensuring effective communication that fosters mutual understanding of goals and procedures.

THE STORY OF LIA LEE

The story of Lia Lee so far has been one of cultural confusion and conflict. Lia's situation had now reached a crisis point. Her original health care providers could no longer manage her care, and the facility was inadequate to the challenge presented by her increasingly complicated problems. Those problems were exacerbated by the difficulties inherent in the cultural complexity of the situation.

Lia Lee was transferred to a children's intensive care unit in Fresno. Her primary physician in Merced explained the transfer as necessary because of her specialized treatment needs and he felt the parents understood; the Lees, however, thought he was transferring her so he could go on vacation. During her lengthy stay at the hospital in Fresno, her parents stayed in the waiting room because they had no money for a hotel. Friends brought them food while they waited. Because Lia was in intensive care, they were not permitted to stay with her, as they had throughout all her previous hospitalizations.

At Fresno, an array of interventions was tried, all without attempt at discussion with her parents because of the language and cultural barriers. Lia was placed on antibiotics, even though a bacterial infection that was probably at the root of the current set of seizures was not diagnosed for several days, and she was anesthetized in an attempt to stop the seizures. She was given oxygen and put on an intravenous line to replace fluids lost through the massive diarrhea caused by the infection. To assist in diagnosis, a spinal tap was performed.

This last procedure was deeply troubling to her father. He felt that "They just sucked her backbone like that and it makes me disappointed and sad because that is how Lia was lost" and "They just took her to the hospital and they didn't fix her. She got very sick and I think it is because they gave her too much medicine" (Fadiman, 1997, p. 148). Although the staff informed the Lees of the procedures through an interpreter, the parents did not understand what was being done to Lia. The terms used were incomprehensible to them. Within a couple of days, Lia was in a vegetative state.

Her former foster mother, Dee Korda, described the scene she encountered when she went to visit the family with Jeanine, the social worker: "It was awful. The doctors wouldn't even look at Foua and Nao Kao. They'd only look at us and Jeanine. They saw us as smart and white, and as far as they were concerned the Lees were neither" (p. 151). Through a translator, the staff informed the Lees that Lia was going to die and then withdrew the intravenous fluids.

Foretelling death is taboo among the Hmong. The Lees felt that the staff was saying that Lia *should die*. They decided to take Lia from the hospital against medical advice. They were convinced that the hospital was mistreating her and that they could provide better care. The staff sent her home in a "persistent vegetative state," convinced that she would die immediately. However, her chart noted that her chief presenting problem, epilepsy, was "resolved."

Summarized from Fadiman, A. (1997). *The spirit catches you and you fall down*. New York: Noonday Press.

INTRODUCTION

The relevance of cultural information for health care focuses on three major questions: What do you need to know? How can you best obtain that information? How does that information shape goals and intervention strategies? In intercultural interactions, gathering and using information to ensure outcomes desired by the client is particularly challenging. As Kim (1996) has noted, "Those who are seriously engaged in direct, face-to-face encounters with people of differing identities are likely to be challenged to change at least some of their internalized cultural assumptions and practices in thinking, feeling, and acting" (p. 356). Such experiences result in what Kim has labeled "**stretching**" for all parties in the interaction. As we have already established, all interactions, even with people who appear very similar to you, will have elements of intercultural interaction; thus, they all present challenges to personal beliefs as well as to established professional guidelines.

We have described culture emergent as a way to conceptualize your client's culture and your own.

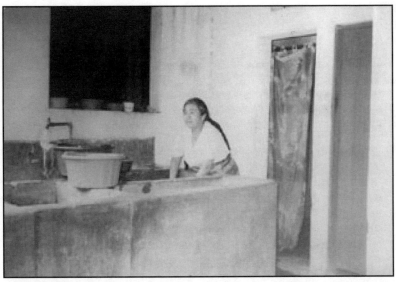

Figure 7-1. Laundry is washed in the family's *pila* in Guatemala.

We have suggested that ethnographic methods can help you understand your vantage and that of your client, as well as reach acceptable mutual cultural accommodations. Here we discuss how these strategies can work in clinical encounters.

It is helpful to remember Sue's (2000) claim described in Chapter 1, that there are three important characteristics for providers who engage in effective intercultural intervention: scientific-mindedness, dynamic sizing skills, and culture-specific expertise. Scientific-mindedness reflects the active curiosity we described earlier. It requires the generation of hypotheses to be tested and modified through careful data collection. Dynamic sizing skills require practitioners to recognize when to generalize about cultural issues and when specific information is needed. Culture-specific expertise requires the acquisition of cultural information for the culture at hand to be used as a base from which to learn about the culture emergent of the individual. These characteristics enable providers to know and understand their clients' cultural groups, the environments in which they live, and the intervention techniques useful to working with such clients. Sue concurs with our contention that it is impossible to know everything about every culture but suggests that providers can know their own values well, undertake careful assessment that includes understanding the probable sources of discrimination for the client, recognize the limits of their knowledge of the client, generate and test hypotheses, attend to their own credibility as well as to any discomfort they experience in the interaction, and actively seek assistance or consultation if needed. He suggests that health care providers who have this mind-set have a higher probability of success with a wide range of individuals than do those who do not.

7-1. Reread the vignette about Lia Lee's transfer to Fresno. How did the health team at Fresno fail to achieve each of Sue's three suggested characteristics?

Q

DETERMINING WHAT YOU NEED TO KNOW

Part of what you need to know is directed by the philosophy and goals of your specific profession. Physicians seek information about physical symptoms and biological change to determine what medicines and other biological interventions might minimize symptoms or cure disease. Physical therapists direct their attention to issues of physical strength, mobility, and endurance. Occupational therapists emphasize the ability to accomplish needed and desired life tasks. Dieticians are concerned almost exclusively with nutrition and habits around food; social workers are interested in the family and larger social setting in which the client lives. Both speech therapists and psychologists are attentive primarily to verbal communication, but with very different goals: speech therapists focus on verbal communication as a physical skill, whereas psychologists use verbal communication techniques to explore feelings and attitudes, self-awareness, and insight. By now it should be evident that cultural factors can affect each of these areas of focus and the questions they require. For example, how much and

MARINA FROM KIEV

Marina is an immigrant from Kiev, Ukraine to Milwaukee, WI. She and her husband left Kiev because they are Jewish and felt the anti-Semitism there was unbearable. Her husband, with the help of a Jewish Family Service Agency social worker, quickly found work in Milwaukee. He developed a group of friends on the job and began to learn English. Meanwhile, Marina has been unable to find work in the 2 years since they moved to the United States. She speaks little English and interacts almost exclusively with her husband. The social worker has continued to visit and has found that Marina spends most of her time reading or sitting alone. When the social worker visits, she tries to point out positive aspects of Marina's current situation, complimenting her on her lovely apartment and furnishings. Marina responds by apologizing for the small apartment, poor furnishings, and meager snacks that she can provide.

- Based on this information, do you think the social worker might believe Marina has a health condition? If so, what diagnosis do you think the social worker might make?

- In Ukrainian culture, it is considered unseemly to show pride in one's possessions. When complimented, it is expected that one will disparage one's belongings. Does this change your view of the social worker's assessment of Marina's current situation?

- Consider for a moment the possibility that the social worker's assessment is accurate but is also mediated by Marina's culturally based responses to the intervention. Has it ever happened in your own experience that you and your physician had differing views about a health condition, and that both of you were partly right?

what kind of mobility is needed (Figure 7-1)? Does the client need to climb trees? Sit on the floor? Walk over cobblestones? Does the diet consist of hamburgers or corn and beans? Does the extended family expect to provide primary support services for the person or to hire someone else to do so?

Q   7-2. Think more about the philosophy and goals of the various professions just mentioned. Identify some potentially culturally variable questions you might need to ask in order to meet each profession's goals.

The other part of what you need to learn requires developing the clearest possible picture of the culture emergent of the individual. Thus, what you need to know includes cultural aspects of daily life and the construction of the current illness or disability (see the box above for an example). How does the general cultural context affect the patient's health status, the evaluation of that status, and the general sense of well-being? What beliefs does the individual have about his or her current health situation? What is the client's individual perception of his or her reasons for needing the intervention? Is the condition assumed to be the result of pulled muscles? Excessive exposure to hot or cold? Angry spirits? Perhaps most importantly, what matters to the person? Mattingly (1998) notes that health care

providers "must address the problem of motivation. They must tap into commitments and values deep enough within patients to commit them to such a process [of health care intervention]" (p. 79). Johnson, Hardt, and Kleinman (1995) indicate that practitioners must know how culture influences illness behavior, determine when cultural differences are important, elicit explanatory models for symptoms, and recognize common ethnic explanatory models.

As an example, think about the possible cultural constructions of suffering. In some cultures, current suffering is perceived as unimportant, as current existence is conceptualized as preparatory to an afterlife in which suffering will be rewarded. In others, current suffering is perceived as the result of misdeeds, either in previous lives or earlier in this life. In still other cultures, suffering simply is what it is, without reference to past or future, to good behavior or bad. Clearly, willingness to engage in treatment may be influenced by these beliefs. If the client believes suffering plays an important role in his or her future life, he or she may be less eager to remediate the causes of the suffering.

Health care and social service providers are concerned about more than their clients' state of physical health. As Radomski (1995) has noted, "there's more to life than putting on your pants" (p. 487), and increasingly, care providers are focused on quality of life or subjective well-being. **Subjective** well-being is the term used to reflect individual perceptions of positive events and level of happiness, and is defined in terms of personal internal experience (Diener, Suh, & Oishi, 1997). *The International Classification of Impairment, Disability, and Handicap* (2nd Edition) terminology for rehabilitation specialists (World Health Organization, 2000) focuses not only on body systems and function, but on activity, participation, and environment with an eye toward enhancing the individual's sense of well-being. The classification system makes clear that activity, participation, and environment all differ across cultures but suggests that by focusing intervention efforts at these three levels, well-being can be enhanced.

Suh, Diener, Oishi, and Triandis (1997) found that judgments about subjective well-being differ across cultures. The degree of correlation between self-esteem and life satisfaction was lower in collectivistic nations than in individualistic ones. Suh et al. (1997) speculate that this finding is because the latter are more likely to emphasize autonomy and internal feelings. They conclude that culture is one of many contextual factors that changes the meaning of experiences and events for the individual. Thus, it is important for care providers to understand the individual's construction of subjective well-being and its correlates, because it is the individual's perceptions that will ultimately determine outcomes. The individual who believes his or her current suffering will lead to a better future life may experience the greatest subjective well-being while experiencing discomfort, whereas another individual who does not hold this belief may want immediate relief. Such differences in evaluation of subjective well-being are essential information for care providers, as they ultimately will affect the care recipient's evaluation of intervention.

It is not just the individual's culture that is important but also the social structure of the culture. Family and social environment affect outcomes. Family structure is a function of culture. Thus, such issues as who makes the decisions can vary from group to group (DiversityRx, 1997b). For some Hispanic families, the grandmother makes health-related decisions even though the father is head of the family for other kinds of decisions (Kreps & Kunimoto, 1994). Such gender differences in family responsibility are common both in the United States and elsewhere but are not identical across cultures. Another example of cultural difference in social structure can be found in family willingness to provide support and care. Among Pueblo Indian caregivers, individual concerns were perceived as less important than issues that might create strains in the extended family (Hennessy & John, 1995). In Japan, public expression about caregiving is positive but may mask underlying negative

THE ALZHEIMER ASSOCIATION

The staff of an urban chapter of the Alzheimer Association observed that although the surrounding community had a large population of African-American individuals, very few of them made use of association support groups, respite care, or caregiver education services. Staff members were puzzled, because they had dramatically increased their service to other groups in the community and had been told by many of those individuals that their services were extremely helpful. At a community leaders' luncheon, the executive director of the association happened to sit next to the pastor from one of the local African-American churches. The director took the opportunity to mention the problem to the pastor. The pastor explained that the African-American community felt strongly about looking after its own older adults in family contexts. He noted that elders are particularly valued and important in inner-city African-American communities because of the support they provide to others. He also indicated that successful interventions by more formal health care systems were usually church-sponsored. The pastor offered to have the executive director come to a church service, at which the pastor described the services offered. Service use in the African-American community immediately increased.

- Based on what you have read in previous chapters, what reasons can you identify for reluctance by members of the African-American community to use formal services?
- What strategy did the executive director use that could be helpful in other situations as well?

attitudes (Koyano, 1989). Health care providers must be concerned with the cultural environment of the individual, as well as his or her own unique characteristics as demonstrated in the boxes on page 133 and below.

CULTURALLY RELEVANT ASSESSMENT

Care providers must obtain accurate, comprehensive information that includes description of cultural characteristics. Traditionally, information has been obtained through administration of interviews and various standardized assessments to measure the attributes of interest. Physicians assess biological systems; social workers evaluate financial and social support. Occupational therapists assess ability to dress, bathe, and engage in leisure activities and work; speech therapists evaluate ability to communicate. Psychologists determine cognitive abilities and the presence of psychological problems; dieticians focus on nutritional status. As soon as culture is factored into the assessment process, specific issues arise in the use of each of these various types of assessments.

Q 7-3. Reflect for a moment on your own profession. What areas of health are the particular focus of your discipline? What factors do you need to know about to begin to plan intervention in those areas?

A recurrent issue is the perceived power relationship between clinician and client. Clients recognize themselves to be dependent on the clinician, and may therefore provide information that they believe to be "what the clinician wants." Their fear of abandonment if they reveal their "real" feelings is a challenge to be overcome. Economic and status differences can have significant impact on the extent to which the client feels comfortable with the provider (Hughes & Okpaku, 1998). Likewise, health care workers may fail to recognize the extent to which they are perceived as power figures, and make inaccurate assumptions about the depth of the client's trust or mistrust. Compounding dilemmas of power is the issue of gender difference. Not only do cultures vary in the ways they ascribe gender roles, they also differ in their view of the appropriate relationship with a care provider of the same or different gender. Health professionals must recognize that within some cultures, certain questions are simply not appropriately put by a man to a woman and vice versa. Whatever one's personal views about gender equality, they must be set aside in the assessment and intervention process. For example, in traditional Mexican families, the man is the decision-maker. A mother may bring her child to a clinic for care, but she may defer any decisions about care to her husband, possibly even delaying needed care to obtain approval from him. For many professional women raised in Old American culture, such a delay would be inexplicable and possibly offensive. Such attitudes would need to be set aside to ensure

---

AN UNCOOPERATIVE YOUNG MAN

One difficult patient was a 25-year-old upper-class Iranian named Hamid Sadeghi. He was very uncooperative and refused to do anything for himself. He would ring for the nurses and demand, "You get here right now and do this." He would not, however, accept anything he had not specifically requested, including lunch trays and medication. He posted a sign on his door that read, "Do not enter without knocking, including the nurses." His attitude caused a great deal of resentment among the nurses (Galanti, 1997).

- What are some possible explanations for Mr. Sadeghi's behavior? Of the explanations you identify, which have a basis in culture, which in individual personality, and which in the situation?

- It is not noted in the description above, but it is possible that the nurses were all female. How might this have affected the patient's behavior, given what you know of his cultural background?

- Although such behavior is offensive to staff, they are still responsible for care of the patient. How might the nurses cope with their feelings of resentment?

that the child received the needed care in the context of his or her own culture and family structure.

Standardized Instruments

Standardized assessments are highly problematic (Rogler, 1999). Even those that seem the most objective, such as manual muscle tests and range of motion tests, have cultural biases. Use of professional terminology ("Is your range of motion limited?" or "Do you limit your activities because of fear of falling?") may lead to misunderstanding. What is meant by range of motion? By fear of falling? Rogler discusses the Diagnostic Interview Schedule for Children, Version 2, a test designed to assess such psychological constructs as anxiety. One question reads: "Do you worry a lot about having clean clothes?" The question assumes that the individual has access to running water and soap. Rogler notes that when the test was administered to a group of Indian adolescents in a Northern Plains community, much worry about clean clothes was discovered. The matter did not have to do with anxiety, however. Rather, it had to do with the difficulties associated with getting laundry done. Differences in perception can easily lead to inaccurate results on these kinds of measures.

Christine Miracle (1981) administered the *Escala de Inteligencia para Niños* to Aymara children in Bolivia who were bilingual in Aymara and Spanish. The *Escala* is a translation of the Wechsler Intelligence Scale for Children (WISC) developed in Puerto Rico but used widely in many Spanish-speaking countries. A host of overt and covert problems were documented by Miracle. The overt problems were primarily language-based, while the covert ones centered on differences in cultural heritages between those for whom the tests were initially intended and those for whom the tests are eventually used. In this case that meant from American English to Puerto Rican Spanish to Bolivian Spanish; and from white middle-class children in the United States through Puerto Rico to rural-oriented poor Native American children in Bolivia.

Language is sometimes a problem in the use of standardized instruments. A practitioner interacting with an individual whose first language is not English may find communication difficult because of vocabulary limitations. In situations where the client speaks no English, the problem is compounded. We discussed in Chapter 5 the idea that translators can help, and, in fact, that use has often been recommended as a strategy. However, use of interpreters is not necessarily sufficient to ensure accurate information-gathering. Spanish is now widely spoken in the United States, but as we have already described, Cuban, Puerto Rican, Mexican, Andean, and Central American Spanish are significantly different, just as British, Australian, and American English are different. A word used to represent a concept in one form of Spanish may not convey the same idea in another as in the examples in the box below. A translator may not have the cultural and linguistic information to recognize the failure of communication. "Translations are fraught with potential errors" (Rogler, 1999, p. 428).

Vocabulary differences are only a small part of language differences. Many of the most significant language differences are matters of usage. A Puerto Rican friend was recently introduced to several Guatemala Mayans. Striving to demonstrate friend-

SAME WORD, DIFFERENT MEANINGS; SAME MEANING, DIFFERENT WORDS IN SPANISH

Word	Meaning	Where
Sobremesa	Tablecloth	Guatemala
	After-dinner conversation	Spain
Pieza	Piece or part	Spain
	Theatrical play	Mexico
	Room	Argentina
Autobús	Bus	Spain
Camión	Bus	Mexico
Camioneta	Bus	Guatemala

ship and solidarity, he immediately addressed them in Spanish, using the familiar form of "you"—*tú*. He was unaware that Spanish used among Mayans is much more formal and that *tú* is used only rarely. Even adult children are addressed by the more formal form of "you"—*usted*. Although a translator can assist with language, the care provider must ask careful questions to ensure that accurate understanding has occurred.

Even when the translator is of the same culture as the individual, misunderstanding can occur because of differing belief systems. A second-generation Mexican American might have adopted many Old American views about health and healing. When translating for a newly immigrated individual who describes himself or herself as suffering from *mal de ojo* (evil eye), the translator might feel that he or she is being asked to describe a fictional, or even ridiculous, condition. The translator might be tempted to maintain his or her own image as a sophisticated, knowledgeable individual by altering the patient's words, creating misunderstanding in both directions in the interaction.

In health care settings, law requires that translators be provided. Title VI of the 1964 Civil Rights Act was the first of a number of bills passed requiring provision of translators as a way to ensure access to health care for all individuals (Office of Minority Health, 2000). There is no question that availability of translators is helpful in many situations; however, clinicians must recognize the limitations inherent in translation.

Gestures also convey meaning. As with language, those meanings are locally defined. Motioning to a client to "come here" could be offensive if, as is true in some cultures, the gesture is used primarily to call animals rather than people. The "thumbs up" gesture used in the United States to wish someone good luck or to indicate approval is deeply offensive to individuals from Iran, where

an identical gesture means essentially "screw you." Clinicians may be tempted to use gestures to convey meaning when talking with someone whose English is limited or absent. This is a logical strategy, but its limitations and risks for misunderstanding must be recognized.

7-4.   A hearing-impaired young man was told that he had tested positive for HIV. He was delighted with this result because in sign language, as in spoken language, "positive" means good. He assumed that the nurse was telling him that he did not have HIV, whereas the nurse was informing him that he did have the virus. What might the nurse have observed that would have let her know there had been a misunderstanding? How could she have gone about clarifying her meaning?

Q

Besides language, there is an issue of interpretation and acceptance of constructs being measured. Cultures have varying beliefs and interpretations about proper behavior that make some mainstream American concepts seem puzzling. For example, one of us administered the Life Satisfaction Inventory (Neugarten, Havighurst, & Tobin, 1961) to several Guatemala Mayans. The interaction resulted in puzzled looks, and ultimately gales of laughter from the Mayans, who could not comprehend questions that asked them to compare their current lives to their past, or themselves to others. They simply did not make these kinds of comparisons. There is a cultural reluctance to make such comparisons because they could invoke strong emotions that could be dangerous. Jealousy, for example, is considered a cause of illness.

Many standardized instruments, even those specifically developed for use across cultures, have similar problems. When the World Health Organization designed the World Health

CULTURAL EXPERIENCE AND STANDARDIZED ASSESSMENTS

Rogler (1999) cites the example of a question on the Dissociative Experience Scale. One question asks how often the individual has had the following experience: "Some people have the experience of driving a car and suddenly realizing that they don't remember what has happened during all or part of the trip" (p. 427). Rogler notes that for inner-city individuals from cultural minorities, long car trips may be rare; such a question would not have meaning for these individuals.

QUESTIONS FROM STANDARDIZED INSTRUMENTS

From the Short Form–36 test (Ware, Snow, Kosinski, & Gandek, 1993):

How much bodily pain have you had during the past 4 weeks?

   None

   Very mild

   Mild

   Moderate

   Severe

   Very severe

From the Satisfaction with Life Scale (Pavot & Diener, 1993):

Rate on a scale from 1 (strongly agree) to 5 (strongly disagree):

So far I have gotten the important things I want in life.

- Consider the two examples. What information do you think they are seeking?
- Compare your answers with those of a classmate or colleague. Did you agree about the nature of the information being sought?
- Now imagine that you are asking for reaction to these items from an inner-city African-American adolescent. How do you think such an individual might interpret these questions? What about a recent Russian immigrant? An elderly Appalachian woman?
- Remember the discussion in this and earlier chapters about cultural interpretation of pain. How might those cultural differences influence responses to the question on the Short Form–36? Might those differences also influence responses on the Satisfaction with Life Scale?

Organization Quality of Life–10, an instrument designed to measure quality of life across cultural groups (Power, Bullinger, Harper, & The WHO Quality of Life Group, 1999), significant efforts to establish satisfactory psychometric attributes across cultures were only moderately successful. Although the researchers found that there are probably universal aspects of quality of life across the 15 cultures they tested, they found differences as well as similarities. Thus, even for instruments that claim cross-cultural validity, interpretation for cultural groups and individuals within those groups must be made cautiously.

Careful examination of instruments and findings may help identify instruments that have utility for particular groups, as well as those for which they are inappropriate (Sullivan et al., 1995). For example, quick screening for literacy can identify individuals whose responses on other standardized instruments are likely to be compromised by inability to read at the needed level. Instruments that have been analyzed using item response theory may provide guidance about differential response by cultural groups (Ellis & Kimmel, 1992), although they may provide little information about individual conformity to those group response patterns.

Norm references are often invalid for cross-cultural comparison. If the goal is to determine where an individual fits in comparison to others, comparison with American college students (a typical normative group for test development) may not be of particular value. If the goal is the more ambiguous comparison with "normal," the problem is in definition of normal. Even among people who are similar, perceptions of normality vary. Add cultural constructs and comparisons become impossible. For example, the Hopi Indians have a classification system for "sicknesses or things that can be wrong with people's minds or spirits" (cited in Rogler, 1999, p. 426). Although seemingly similar to the Old American construction of depression, the Hopi classification system has been found to have no direct analog, leading to inaccurate diagnosis in this population.

THE ADOPTED SALVADORAN GIRL

A young girl was adopted from El Salvador by an American family. The family, motivated by altruism and a belief that such an adoption was an important humanitarian service, nonetheless made assumptions about the abilities of the child. They were therefore dismayed to discover when she arrived in their home that, at age 10, she ate with her hands and seemed undisciplined and uncommunicative. Similarly, her teachers in the semi-rural, affluent suburb where the family lived found her unable to behave in a fashion they considered appropriate. She did not respond to lessons, did not pay attention, and almost never spoke or responded to questions. A speech therapist with some college Spanish evaluated her and concluded that she was developmentally delayed. Another teacher suggested an outside evaluation by a cultural specialist. A consultant was called in, preparatory to placing the child in a special education class.

- Take a moment to consider this example. What are some alternative explanations for the girl's behavior? What additional information would you need to determine what was really occurring? What are some approaches you could use to obtain the information?

If you were in the situation, it would be important to determine some precise information about the child's background culture. What is the dominant language? What are child-rearing practices like? What are the expectations for childhood behavior? What are the characteristics of the physical environment? Such information might be obtained from knowledgeable informants, from the literature, and from Internet searches.

In this case, the consultant happened to be familiar with the culture from which the girl had come. The consultant spent time simply observing the child. Because she came to the situation with a particular knowledge set, she was able to generate alternative explanations for the behavior. The consultant realized, for example, that prior to coming to the United States, the child had probably never seen a fork. She spoke no English and used a regional form of Spanish, nothing like what is taught in American college courses. Thus, she did not understand the instructions she was given, and could not respond in an effective fashion. It became clear that her "developmental delay" was primarily a result of lack of exposure to English and a frustrating inability to communicate effectively. The consultant pointed out that no one in the child's new environment could even pronounce her name correctly. These problems were not likely to be remedied in a special education classroom. In fact, the consultant found the child, speaking comfortably in Spanish, to be verbal, articulate, curious, and even witty. A sort of mutual accommodation was required in this situation, in which parents and teachers made the effort to find more effective ways to communicate and initial behavioral expectations were matched more closely with the girl's prior experience.

- What type of activities might you suggest for the parents and teachers of this child?
- How might they enhance their ability to communicate with her?

Some norm-referenced instruments may have utility as a means to determine an individual's abilities in a way that can then be measured against a culturally meaningful standard. For example, it may not matter how a woman's strength compares with that of other women her age, but it may matter whether she has the strength it takes to hoe a field. It may not matter whether a man is more sad or less sad than other men his age, but it may matter whether he is too sad to be able to mobilize himself for work in the morning.

Gathering culturally relevant information is no small challenge. However, effective outcomes depend on the skill with which such information is obtained. People may be unaccustomed to discussing the importance of emotions or activities in their lives, or the meaning those feelings and activities hold for them.

Adoption can be fraught with such dilemmas even when there is an expectation of similarity. For example, many prospective parents prefer to adopt from countries like Russia, where the children will appear similar to them. A colleague shared a story about a trip she took to Russia to assist a couple who was adopting an infant. The colleague noted with dismay that among mothers in Russia who gave up their children for adoption, alcoholism was a significant concern. Further, once the children were placed in an orphanage to await adoption, their environment was unstimulating. The many toys that had been sent or brought by adoptive parents were kept behind a partition so that the toys "would not be spoiled." The parents expected a normal, healthy 6-month-old baby; the clinician observed an infant with signs of fetal alcohol syndrome and sensory deprivation syndrome.

Q   7-5.   What reactions might you expect from the parents as they learn that their child has an array of developmental problems?

7-6.   What might the therapist do to help the parents adjust their expectations?

Clinicians must bear in mind that cultural issues are present in every assessment situation. Wohl (1989) has speculated that they may actually be most intense in those situations in which the provider seems most like the client. He notes that in these situations, the potential for making inaccurate assumptions and for failing to gather relevant information is great because of the perception that the two are "alike."

Ethnographic Interviewing in the Clinical Setting

Culturally relevant assessment can be pursued using **qualitative methods**, as we described in Chapters 5 and 6. Although there are some constraints (primarily time), qualitative strategies can provide meaningful data regarding the interplay of culture with the current health situation of the individual. Bruner (1987) suggests viewing "**life as narrative**" (i.e., understanding individuals through the stories they tell about their lives and experiences). Use of **qualitative interviewing** can provide access to information that allows clinicians to "articulate and enter into the [client's] subjective world view" (McClure & Teyber, 1996, p. 5).

Rubin and Rubin (1995) define qualitative interviews as similar to ordinary conversations, differing largely in terms of intensity of listening to what is said. The essential element is careful listening for meaning. This practice includes listening sentence by sentence and word by word, with the goal of getting to "thick description" (Geertz, 1984) of the individual's personal experiences. Such description is rich with detail and elaboration that enhances the interviewer's understanding of the

perspective of the individual.

Effective qualitative interviewing requires empathy, sensitivity, humor, and sincerity. The interviewer must recognize his or her own biases and beliefs but must also be willing to acknowledge that "one person's experiences are not intrinsically more true than another's" (Rubin & Rubin, 1995, p. 10). The interviewer must bring to the interview not only an awareness of possible personal biases, but also at least some understanding of culture generally and, ideally, some specific information about the culture of the individual. Such an interview involves active listening rather than frequent questioning, as the interviewer makes an effort to understand the client's vantage on the problem at hand and his or her life circumstances.

Specific Interview Strategies

Interview strategies vary somewhat depending on the information being sought. The overall strategy is to design a flexible, iterative, and continuous series of questions that seek to obtain the individual's world view, rather than a set of general statements about a particular culture. The general pattern for such an interview would be as follows:

- Clarify your purpose. Ask permission. "I would like to interview you about the pain in your arm when you make tortillas so I can see if I can help you do this better. May I ask you some questions?"

- Let the client know that she or he has permission to decide against answering questions; however, do not assume that the client will always take advantage of this permission. Clients who perceive themselves as having very low status, or being very dependent on your help, may fear the consequences if they refuse. You must be especially sensitive to signs of discomfort, weariness, or embarrassment, including facial grimaces, shift in gaze, shift in body position, and so on.

- Depending on the situation, the assessment itself might start with a very general question ("Why are you here today?") or an extremely specific one ("Where does it hurt?").

- Ask several follow-up questions to obtain greater depth of understanding. For example, "Could you give me an example of...?" or "What is the effect of...?"

- Ask for clarification. "What do you mean by...?" "I did not understand what you told me about X. Please tell me more."

- Ask for temporal clarification. "What do you do first?" "How does this fit into your day?"
- Request details. "How do you...?"
- Ask questions you think may be stressful or highly personal later in the interview, carefully monitoring reactions. If the person appears uncomfortable, or avoids answering, change the subject and come back to it. It can be helpful to explain exactly why such information is required. If you cannot explain it, perhaps you do not really need it.
- Observe carefully. Watch for differences between verbal response and behavior. Such differences might suggest that the question was not understood or that the individual is unable or unwilling to provide accurate verbal information. Many individuals feel intimidated in health care encounters and are concerned with providing the "right" or "expected" information. Particularly in situations where future care or placement decisions might hinge on responses, verbalizations may be carefully chosen. Once they discovered that their responses could result in removal of their child from their home, for example, the Lee family might have been much more reticent about providing accurate information.
- Remember that reality is in the eye of the beholder and is not static. According to Mattingly (1998), a large body of literature suggests that reality is constructed through the telling of stories (i.e., through narrative that reflects personal interpretation, the making of meaning from a series of events).
- Keep careful notes. Practice the system described in Chapter 5 by which you can capture detailed information quickly so that you can review and ask follow-up or clarification questions at a later time. As much as possible, capture word choice, tone, and body posture, as well as the content of the response.

As you ask questions, you are listening carefully for word choice, for hesitation, for body language, for contradiction. Even if you think you understand what the client has said, ask the question in several different ways. Tell the client what you think was said and ask for confirmation. Over time, work toward identifiable themes that might explain the client's perceptions. As you develop these themes, check them repeatedly with the client to ensure that your view accurately represents his or her view. Your goal is to learn about the client's vantage. How

does the client see the world and the current problem? What resources does the client feel are available? From the client's vantage, what additional resources are needed?

7-7. Consider the example interview segment on pages 141-142. Try to identify the ways in which the interviewer followed each of our suggested interview strategies.

7-8. Interview someone you know—a classmate, a family member, a coworker, a neighbor—on one of the following topics for 20 minutes, using the strategies described above. If possible, tape the interview; in any case, take careful notes.
- What are your beliefs about friendship?
- Describe someone you admire tremendously, either a historical figure or someone living today.
- Describe in detail the most important activity in your life and why it is so important to you.

7-9. How did you prepare for this interview? What was the most difficult part for you? What seemed to be the most difficult part for your interviewee? Would you change anything the next time you interview someone?

In the process of asking questions, it is important to demonstrate respect for the individual. Although you enter the assessment with a certain amount of already ascribed credibility as a clinician, you must also achieve credibility through your interactions (McClure & Teyber, 1996). Health care professionals are often encouraged to establish rapport with their clients. Rapport-building is not a quick process that can be accomplished through an introductory statement. However, thoughtful introductory interactions are essential to beginning the process. Always introduce yourself and your purpose. Check the individual's understanding of that purpose through your interaction. Determine the individual's preferred manner of address, both for him- or herself and for you. You might be most comfortable with a first-name basis, but the client might not be.

Recognize that these steps are only a beginning. It is unreasonable and unrealistic to assume that once you have been introduced, the individual will inevitably trust you. You are, after all, likely to

A Sample Interview

This interview was part of an ethnographic study of older, community-residing women. The research participant is classified as an Old American—a white, Lutheran woman, whose family originally emigrated from Germany at the beginning of the 19th century. Now widowed, she is a mother of six, grandmother of nine. She is retired from a clerical job with a small suburban government, and is living alone in a small bungalow near four of her grown children. Segments presented here are from the preliminary portion of the interview, focused on demographic and historical information, and from the section in which her religious beliefs and practices are being explored (I = the interviewer, P = the client).

I: Tell me a little about your parents.

P: They're both dead. My mother died in '82, my father died in '88.

I: Where did your parents live?

P: They lived in Minnesota, in a little town there.

I: Is that where they were born?

P: Yes, they had a big extended family there, but I don't see them much. They're all old or have died, so there are very, very few. I moved away a long time ago.

I: I'd like to know more about the town where you were raised. What was it like being a small child there?

P: We all worked really hard. My father had a farm a little way from town, and we had to help all the time. My brother went out with my father, and the girls helped at home. My father didn't really like farming, and he wasn't too good at it. He didn't think we should farm, but he didn't know what we could do. It was really a tiny town. I guess it was OK.

I: When did you move away?

P: When I was... uh, 19. War was declared, and, uh, I was going to school, and they said that you have this chance, we'll send you, this was when Pearl Harbor, right after, you can go to Washington, DC to work. I was raised on a farm and very poor, poor, and, uh, I, and my mother, I can't imagine my mother, I would not let my girls do this, or would not encourage it. I got on a train knowing nobody, knowing not where I was going to stay or anything... but my father didn't like girls that much... oh, well, you know, he really loved me I'm sure, but he thought girls should just work on the farm...

I: How about brothers and sisters?

P: I've got a brother that thinks, uh, he's got a dachshund—he never married—that is worth a million dollars. Stuff like that. So no, I've talked to him on the phone, but I have not, or saw him last year and that's... so I don't really see them that much. I'm really very unrelated to my family because I've been gone so long, leaving at 19 you know, your life does not revolve around that part of your family.

I: Your parents' families originally came from Germany. Is that right?

P: Yeah.

I: And so did your family keep any German traditions?

P: Well, we eat really heavy food. I worry about my cholesterol now and can't believe I ate all of that. You know, pork chops and potatoes and fried chicken. Really bad. But we, I don't know, we didn't seem really German. Our Christmas was German, I guess. But the church was more important. We went to the Lutheran church, and my life has always centered around the church. I'm very involved in the church.

I: Clearly church is a real central focus of your life. Can you tell me more about it?

P: I was born in the Lutheran area of Minnesota and I went to parochial school. I, when I was working for the war department, I never, never left the church, never. I never left the church. I probably, I probably in my life have missed only maybe 30 Sundays. Oh, and no, it's, there's just no... I go to church every Sunday, and it's just been a vital part of my life.

I: How are you involved in the church? Is this primarily through going to services?

continued

P: Well, uh, I always go to services, but there's other things, too. Our president of the congregation was a Christian woman president and I get I think you know desperate desperation, nobody wants to be it and I after, so I became president and I've got until May and then I'm out but I'm on the board...

I: So what else do you do at church?

P: Well, I already told you I'm on the board. And, uh, I do a lot of volunteer work with the church, you know, like meals on wheels, and all the other volunteer work. And I go every Sunday, and one day the pastor asked me to do a segment he calls "My walk with the Lord." And I talked about my husband and how I had to nurse him when he was sick. I also give communion every month to, uh, to people in homes, three people right now that I take communion right after the Sunday service... they can't go out, and sometimes I wonder what that would be like, but you just take things as they are. I take things as they come pretty much.

I: When you say that, you take things as they come...

P: When you cannot change what comes.

I: Do you think that's a reflection of your faith? That attitude?

P: Well, right, yeah, it's a reflection, but what, whatever, I should say, whatever God deals to me I take it. Whatever, uh, there's things in life you cannot do a thing about, you know, at all.

I: When you look ahead, what are the things that you feel most invested in, in terms of your activities, the things you do? What are the things that you feel most invested in, and you feel like you really want to be able to do?

P: Church, the church, yeah. You know, I would never, I never miss a Sunday. I'm very involved in the church. And I, I love the church. I've been active a long time, and the church is the church, whoever is the minister, whoever the participants, but that is my church. That's probably where I get to put most of my time.

I: Now, when you talk about the church, you're obviously talking about much more than going to services.

P: Right, I work on the board, and the Bible school, which is a pain working there, 'cause you know you are dealing with a lot of kids, and I take my two grandchildren. Bible school is a whole week of the summer, which is very intense, every day all morning. I work in the kitchen, you know. I help with the suppers. And I take care of the altar with a team.

I: So how big would your team be for this?

P: Four. Three are there all the time, but one drops in and out. So you go there Saturday morning, then you have to be there Saturday night. And twice on Sunday and then on Monday morning.

I: What do you do to take care of the altar?

P: You have to make sure everything is clean, and everything the pastor needs is there, and the flowers are in good shape. And the communion has to be ready. Did I tell you I give communion too?

I: What's that like?

P: They have a nice little chalice, and a thing that holds the wafer, so you just, the ritual of the service of communion, and I do three women once a month and I go to their houses because they can't come to services.

I: And when you're in their homes, you give them communion?

P: Right, and chit-chat, and that's what they really like.

ask relatively intrusive and personal questions, some of which might seem rude or improper to the individual. Careful explanation of your need to know and mechanisms for the individual to decline answering in a graceful way can help establish trust. For example, you might say to the client, "I can help you best if I understand more about any problems with using the bathroom. If you feel uncomfortable about any of the questions I ask, please let me know. Maybe we can figure out some other way to deal with the issue."

Consider this example. A middle-aged man

presented to a clinic for assessment. During the course of a general medical history, the physician asked the client, "Are you sexually active?" The man responded in the affirmative. She then asked, "What kind of contraception do you use?" He hesitated and then said, "I'm gay. That's worked so far."

Q 7-10. What do you think the physician said next? What do you think the client was trying to accomplish?

7-11. How might you yourself respond to such an assertion? What kinds of issues would it raise in terms of your own values and beliefs? In what way is this an example of a cross-cultural encounter?

7-12. What kinds of questions have your physicians or other care providers asked you that made you uncomfortable or made you feel they did not understand you? How might they have put you at ease?

Specific questions will vary naturally depending on the client, the situation, and your own discipline. Kleinman (1980) suggests that physicians ask their patients the following questions:

- What do you call the problem?
- What do you think has caused your problem?
- Why do you think it started when it did?
- What do you think the sickness does? How does it work?
- How severe is the sickness? Will it have a short or a long course?
- What kind of treatment do you think you should receive? What are the most important results you hope to receive from the treatment?
- What are the chief problems that the sickness has caused?
- What do you fear most about the sickness?

Q 7-13. What problems do you see in using these questions in your own professional practice? What modifications might you make to the questions to make them fit more comfortably with your professional culture or practice setting?

7-14. What questions might you omit? What new ones might you add?

Kleinman's questions may not suit the needs of all care providers, but they are an example of how an interview might be structured to obtain information. It is essential to recall that the individual may not be able to provide the needed information. Many of us would have difficulty providing concise summaries about our beliefs regarding health and illness. A useful strategy is to encourage the individual to tell the story in his or her own way. It is your job to discover in the story the information that can guide your intervention.

In clinical settings, you have need for particular kinds of information. Specific questions may be required by regulatory agencies. For example, the Minimum Data Set (MDS), an evaluation required for all nursing home residents covered by Medicare, asks providers to evaluate such factors as "resident believes he/she is capable of increased independence in at least some **Activities of Daily Living**" and "resident makes negative statements" (Health Care Financing Administration, 1999). In many settings, gathering this information is challenging, because the MDS is not designed to incorporate cultural or language issues. In these situations, observation, restatement of questions in different words, and even demonstration and pantomime may yield more valid information.

Unfortunately, time pressure often limits the care provider's ability to use such strategies. Considerable creativity may then be required. Some facilities have developed quick check sheets that permit only a limited number of questions, with three or four response categories that are simply checked off as the evaluation proceeds. The problem with this strategy lies in the severe limits it places on ability to record the breadth and depth of information needed to grasp the individual's circumstances. You may feel more comfortable if you recognize that assessment is a constant, ongoing process, and the information that cannot be obtained within the time constraints of the first assessment may be gathered as interaction continues throughout the intervention process.

INTERVENTION

Goal-Setting

As we have noted, health care professionals are increasingly concerned with various aspects of quality of life and subjective well-being as the ultimate goals of intervention. There is now considerable

ACTIVITY, QUALITY OF LIFE, AND CULTURE

Activity contributes significantly to quality of life and its meaning (Csikszentmihalyi, 1975). Individuals who have valued activities and are able to engage in them will experience high levels of subjective well-being. The choice of activity is highly personal but clearly influenced by cultural norms.

All activity choices and patterns are influenced by culture. Activities of daily living such as cooking, eating, and self-care all have cultural components. For example, in traditional Mayan communities in rural highland Guatemala, preparing a meal involves gathering wood for a fire, building the fire, grinding corn for tortillas, shaping the tortillas, and cooking them on a wood-burning stove. The meal itself is begun and ended with patterned social interaction that is considered an integral part of dining.

- Compare this pattern with your own meal preparation and traditions around the meal itself. Or compare your bed-making routine with that of a Japanese woman who rolls up the futon and moves it out of the center of the floor each morning.

In some societies, individuals have considerable choice about income-generating activities. In industrial societies, individuals may choose to work in factories, on farms, in schools and universities, in health care, or in other arenas. However, individual choice is mediated by environmental and social circumstances. For example, individuals with little education and few skills will have limited choice regarding work. Cultural dictates about the proper roles of men and women may also influence work choices.

When an activity has a strong cultural component, disability can lead to significant decrease in one's own sense of well-being. However, in these cases, individuals may find adaptations. For example, one Mayan woman said that she felt a great loss when arthritis pain made it impossible for her to weave. Because of the rigid cultural rules guiding the weaving activity, she did not perceive modifying the activity as an option. Her husband was a church elder, and she reestablished her identity through ceremonial and social activities associated with his position. She felt that her spiritual, social, and identity needs were addressed through this alternate role.

A weaver in the United States described the consequences of a stroke that left her hemiplegic. Despite this physical impairment, she continued to weave, producing goods that were shown at art shows to much favorable comment. To continue to weave, she had to make a number of modifications in the process, arranging the batten so she could use it with her one good hand and connecting the foot pedals so that she could raise and lower the frames with her one usable foot. This woman was determined to continue to weave and was able to modify the occupation to fit her current abilities.

- Think about an activity that is important in your life. How do you think you would feel if you could no longer do this activity?
- What strategies might you use to deal with the change in your daily life pattern if you could no longer do the activity?
- How do you think those strategies might be different if you were from a culture that had rigid rules about gender-appropriate behavior? About expectations of people with disabilities?

These examples suggest that clinicians must be alert to cultural factors evident in activity and to incorporate them into intervention plans. Recommendations that are in conflict with values and beliefs, or that do not directly address the needs fulfilled by the individual in the context of her or his culture, may be less likely to be successful in remediating the identified problem. Understanding the client's vantage is essential in structuring successful interventions.

evidence that objective health is not strongly correlated with subjective well-being (Okun, Stock, Haring, & Witter, 1984). We know, for example, that people confined to wheelchairs are approximately as happy as those who are not disabled (Allman, 1990). Individuals are able to adapt to such conditions so that even life-altering events, such as spinal cord injury, do not alter subjective well-being over the long term. Within about 8 weeks after their injury, individuals with such injuries report greater pleasant than unpleasant effects (Silver, 1980). Thus, even when the illness or disability cannot be cured, the individual can live a satisfying life.

Many decisions about intervention are driven by quality of life considerations. For example, physicians are routinely confronted with situations in which they must decide about full disclosure of a diagnosis, a circumstance that becomes problematic particularly when the diagnosis is terminal. In Old American culture, beliefs regarding appropriate openness about such diagnoses have changed rapidly, and the widely held view now is that it is essential to be completely open and honest. However, many cultures hold other views (Pimental, Ferreira, Real, Mesquita, & Maia-Goncalves, 1999). In the south and east of Europe and in Japan, it is considered better to withhold the diagnosis to avoid causing the person feelings of hopelessness. Pimental et al. (1999) examined the values of Portuguese individuals and found that disclosure of the diagnosis did not have a negative influence on quality of life. However, in a society in which openness is not valued, it might. All other intervention decisions about how to treat a terminal illness will be influenced by this initial decision.

All clinicians must remember that both culture and individual factors affect intervention plans. A dietitian must be aware that traditional foods vary slightly depending on the skills and preferences of the cook. Physical capacity influences enactment of tasks in every culture. Because of the interplay of environment and activity, in some cultures, physical impairment is much more limiting than in others. For example, where streets are not paved, being in a wheelchair or on crutches can be much more limiting than in areas where sidewalks ease ambulation. This contrast does not always hold, however, because in more communal areas, the individual in a wheelchair may be able to get help from others, whereas in the big city, buildings may be built without regard for accessibility and passers-by may be disinclined to help. Consideration of these factors should influence the ways in which a physical therapist chooses to assist a client in regaining functional mobility.

It is also possible that the most effective intervention may be one that focuses directly on vantage, rather than on health status. Reinterpretation of the story (Mattingly, 1998) may help the individual perceive the functional change in a different manner. For example, John Callahan (1989), a well-known cartoonist, has been quadriplegic for many years since being injured in a serious car accident. However, he describes himself not as a quadriplegic, but as a recovering alcoholic, because in his view, it was his alcoholism that was a disability. After the accident, he focused primarily on treatment for his substance abuse problem, not on physical rehabilitation. Likewise, Robert Murphy (1987), a noted anthropologist, complained about being perceived by his colleagues and therapists as disabled; in his own view, he was able to accomplish all the activities that were important in his life.

There are realistic constraints on the evaluation and intervention processes in health care and social services, compounded by the difficulties of accurately recording and analyzing information obtained and by the complexity of designing intervention strategies that suit the particular culture. With sufficient creativity, it is possible to design strategies specialized to fit unusual circumstances.

Consider the approach used in a refugee camp through which Lia Lee's family passed (Fadiman, 1997). The physician there, Dwight Conquergood, refused to label clients as noncompliant, but rather tried to use traditional beliefs to reach people with new information. Using impromptu theatrical pro-

THE FAMILY IN THE HOSPITAL ROOM

Susie Chung is a 24-year-old Chinese-American woman admitted to the hospital with right lower quadrant abdominal pain. She is taken to surgery for an emergency appendectomy and returns to the floor after having done well in surgery. Her vital signs are good and her prognosis is excellent. The nurse is dismayed to find that Ms. Chung's immediate and extended family fill her room, hovering over her. The nurse finds it difficult to administer nursing care because of the number of family members keeping constant watch (Giger & Davidhizar, 1991).

- What are some reasons Ms. Chung's family might be in her room? What do you think Ms. Chung's response to her family might have been? How could the nurse find out?

- How could the nurse reconsider the situation to deliver necessary care more effectively while respecting the needs and wishes of the patient and family?

ductions featuring characters common in Hmong folk tales, he explained the need to inoculate dogs against rabies, clean latrines, and adopt other health-related behaviors. Clinicians are under time pressure, of course, and are constrained by regulations about intervention. Theatrical productions are beyond typical limits, but perhaps there are other ways to incorporate culture. The inquiring, sensitive, ethnographic mind is always alert to imagine what some of these might be.

To some extent, goal setting and intervention are the ultimate cultural accommodations. The client has begun the process of accommodation by coming to see you in a cultural environment that is likely to feel foreign and perhaps even frightening. The process of negotiating goals that meet the client's needs while also meeting your professional expectations and the constraints of the environment is a process of learning about each other's cultures and determining how those cultures can be made to work together.

Creative clinicians will not only explore mechanisms for culturally relevant interventions, they will also give consideration to mechanisms for moving beyond the limits imposed by their institutions. Where an intervention is not possible in the context of the physical therapy clinic, or in the guidelines for social work interventions, it may be possible to identify someone else in the treatment team who may be able to implement the treatment. For example, the physical therapist might be able to have the health educator plan the theatrical production that is not possible in the physical therapy clinic. Community resources are another avenue for providing interventions that are not within the framework of the health care institution. The social worker may be able to guide the speech pathologist in identifying the community service that can provide the oral reading practice needed by a Spanish-speaking individual following a cerebrovascular accident. A psychologist might try to identify a local community church that can provide social support for a client.

Practitioners must be creative in structuring assessment and intervention while establishing a therapeutic alliance that can be of value to the client. As we observed in the previous chapter, Mattingly (1998) has referred to the concept of "underground practice." Underground practice is practice that addresses a client's other real needs off the records while accomplishing the goals set by third party payers and other regulators. For example, in the United States, most older adults pay for

health care through Medicare, a government-sponsored program. Medicare has strict rules for what it will and will not reimburse. However, some of what it does not reimburse may be most vital to the health and well-being of the individual.

Consider the situation of a 78-year-old woman sent home after 2 weeks of rehabilitation for a broken hip. The woman, a widow, lived alone in a high-rise apartment building with an elevator. Until her accident, she had been driving independently, actively participating in volunteer activities, spending time at movies and restaurants with her large circle of friends, and occasionally looking after her grandchildren. Rehabilitation had prepared her to manage (barely) in her apartment, so that with difficulty she could dress, bathe, and fix a simple meal. It had not addressed any other issues—most notably, her fear and depression about the possible consequences of her physical situation on her ability to continue her outside activities. A home health therapist was sent in to ensure her safety in the apartment, but knew that her services would not be reimbursed if she spent time dealing with the woman's "leisure" activities. Only self-care was reimbursed.

The therapist felt conflicted: her professional culture dictated that she address client needs, but her organizational culture dictated that she provide only reimbursable services. She identified two goals with the woman: increased endurance during ambulation and improved dressing ability. As a means of working on safe ambulation, she and the woman walked to and from her car and then practiced using the foot pedals. In the course of informal discussion while working on dressing, they discussed the accessibility of various buildings in the community. Such strategies do not subvert the rules of the organization, nor do they violate law. Rather, they make the most efficient and creative use of time allotted for intervention.

It is not only underground practice that calls for creativity. Think about the dilemma of the speech therapist working with a Chinese man recovering from a laryngectomy resulting from laryngeal cancer. The electrolarynx typically used in the United States to allow for speech by such individuals creates a monotone sound that cannot begin to communicate the important meanings conveyed by tone in Chinese (DiversityRx, 1997b). The therapist in such a situation must consider alternatives: Can the electrolarynx be reprogrammed? Can hand motions, facial expression, or some other cue substitute for tone? What other options might exist?

STRATEGIES THAT WORK WITHIN TIME CONSTRAINTS

- Remember that every interaction is an opportunity for both assessment and treatment. If your time with the client is limited to 15 minutes, remember that "casual" conversation can provide valuable information. In fact, in many instances, that informal conversation during the course of other activity (e.g., transfer practice, cooking, dressing evaluation) may provide the most useful information because the client may be less focused on giving you the "right" answers. It also serves as an opportunity to disseminate vital information.

- Attend to observed behavior in designing interventions. Where does the patient's spouse sit while being instructed on intervention? If she or he sits on the floor, this suggests that your transfer techniques need to focus on a particular set of strategies to determine where individuals of that culture typically sit and how to facilitate that ability.

- Ask questions, demonstrate techniques, and practice skills more than once. During the course of informal interactions, remember to ask relevant questions repeatedly. Over time, as the client gains confidence in the relationship, answers may be more complete. Repeated discussion will certainly provide richer description. In addition, a modification of wording as you better understand the client's linguistic usage may yield more accurate description. Further, you will begin to identify better the client's actual understanding of the information you are trying to convey.

- Watch carefully for verbal cues to meaning. Pay close attention to pauses, hesitation, change in voice tone, word choice, repetition, and contradictions. Any of these might give you useful information about behavior and beliefs that the client cannot articulate directly. Likewise, they will provide cues to any misunderstanding that has occurred in your communication with the client.

- Note behavioral cues to meaning. Shift in body posture or eye position, increased motor activity, twitches, etc., can be valuable guides to interpretation.

- Check your information. As we have established, it is impossible to know everything about every culture. Even if you could, you would still need to incorporate individual factors. As you gather information and make interpretations, ask for clarification and confirmation. Check your interpretations with the individual, with other cultural informants, and with the literature.

The speech therapist also might have to consider creative intervention strategies with patients such as the elderly Creek Indian woman following a cerebrovascular accident (Orlansky & Heward, 1981). The woman lost most of her speech as a result of the cerebrovascular accident, and when her speech began to return, it was in her native language, not in English.

Q

7-15. What strategies might the therapist try in order to facilitate communication with the patient in the immediate situation?

7-16. How might the therapist approach the longer-term problem of helping the woman to communicate with her family and friends?

Ideally, goals will be negotiated with the client. You may perceive independence in self-care as vital, whereas an older Hispanic client may feel that her children should take care of her. The children, on the other hand, may have acculturated more to the Old American, individualistic perspective, which might reduce their sense of obligation to the older individual. These conflicting perspectives must be addressed in the goal-setting process.

As a strategy for checking the appropriateness of goals, McClure and Teyber (1996) recommend developing a **case conceptualization** based on information about the culture, the environment, and the individual. This case conceptualization, like the example given on page 148, can be checked with the individual and goals compared with the problems identified in that conceptualization. Once goals are agreed upon, strategies for addressing them can be designed.

EXAMPLE CASE CONCEPTUALIZATION

Mrs. Garcia (a pseudonym) sat with her eyes downcast before her four adult children, a family practice resident, and myself, a behavioral scientist. I had been called to help persuade this 62-year-old Hispanic patient to consent to a modified radical mastectomy recommended by a consulting surgeon.

The resident had referred the patient 6 months ago for a biopsy of a right breast mass. The patient had refused the procedure and further health check-ups. Her family eventually persuaded her to consent to the procedure with the surgeon, who then diagnosed an intraductal adenocarcinoma. Now, a modified radical mastectomy was needed, and she was refusing surgery.

The family pleaded, reasoned, and pressured her to have the surgery, but they were unsuccessful. Her family consented to accept her decision if she agreed to speak with her family physician. Why did she refuse surgery? It was not for the obvious reasons: fear of losing a breast, dying during surgery, or suffering the ordeals of chemotherapy. Instead, she stated that she did not need the surgery because she no longer had cancer. She said she had been cured by the prayer vigils held at her home for the last week.

The resident came to me 1 hour before the scheduled family session and asked me for help. I was thinking I had absolutely no idea of how to approach the patient.

The faces of the patient's family told me they were at their wits' end and could only hope that I would think of something. The resident began the session by welcoming everyone. To obtain a good understanding of the course of events, a feel for the patient and family, and more time to think, I asked to review the medical history and events. After the resident spoke, the patient said in a defensive tone to me, "They don't think that I know what I'm talking about. I'm cured; I don't have cancer. My prayer group said that my cancer is cured. The power of the Lord is strong." As she mentioned her prayer group curing her cancer, I could see through the corner of my eye that the family members were shaking their heads and rolling their eyes. In a soft voice, a daughter clarified that the prayer group never claimed to cure the cancer nor did they discourage surgery.

Wanting to further strengthen my alliance with Mrs. Garcia, given that I received this challenging information from the family, I said, "I find you to be clear and strong about what you say and believe. It is good that you have support from your prayer group and faith in God." Proudly and righteously, Mrs. Garcia turned to her family. "You see, he is a doctor and says that I know what I am talking about!"

Now that I had her trust and respect, an idea came to me about how to help her compromise while still maintaining her faith in her God. I did not even give myself time to censor or critique my thoughts. I said to her, "God is powerful, isn't he?" "Yes," she proudly asserted.

"I think we need to reassure the surgeon and your family, who are all worried about you," I said. "Why don't we let the surgeon see for himself that the cancer is gone? If you give him permission to do the surgery, then he could see for himself that the cancer is gone. He and your family would not have to worry." To my surprise, she said, "Yes, that would be all right."

We still had to get consent for the mastectomy. I said, "Now, if by chance the tumor came back as it can sometimes happen, then would you give the surgeon permission to remove the tumor and your breast?" Without reservation she agreed, but added, "I don't want him to remove anything if there is no cancer." I reassured her with, "I know the surgeon well, and I promise that I will call him and let him know that if he does not see a tumor that he should not remove your breast."

The resident hesitantly added that Mrs. Garcia would have to sign a consent form saying that she is consenting to the surgeon removing her breast. I said to Mrs. Garcia, "So you understand that you will have to sign forms stating that you understand that the surgery is done to remove your breast?" "Yes," she said, "As long as he will take nothing off if there is no tumor." I responded, "I will also make sure that if he sees no mass, then he will not remove your breast." She agreed.

I called the surgeon, who often works with our family practice residents, and he agreed that he would acknowledge our discussion and state that if no tumor existed, then he would not remove her breast. The surgery occurred, and the breast cancer was found, and the breast was removed.

continued

She interpreted her need for the mastectomy as due to her cancer coming back. She had an excellent recovery. Two years later, she is traveling, visiting relatives, and still firmly believing in her God.

Mrs. Garcia's claims that she had no cancer expressed not only her faith in her God but also her own strength. She wanted to feel respect through acknowledgment of her beliefs before she could continue making any compromises. I could have challenged her denial of having cancer, but this would have further alienated her from her family and health care providers. Or I could have viewed her position against surgery as expressing her right to die and forego viable treatment options. If Mrs. Garcia had said, "I'd rather live my life without a mastectomy," then I would have defended her wish not to have the surgery. However, through respectful acknowledgment of her belief systems, we were able to achieve a successful outcome.

Zamudio, A. (2000). Finding solutions through the eyes of our patients. *Family Medicine, 32,* 15-16. Reprinted with permission, Society of Teachers of Family Medicine.

DESIGNING INTERVENTIONS WITH CULTURE IN MIND

Sensitivity to Personal Factors in the Context of Culture

Intervention decisions must reflect the individual so both personal and cultural factors must be considered in intervention choice. Remember the young psychologist working in the day treatment center described in Chapter 5. For more than a month, she persisted in her efforts to encourage employment for the program participants. For more than a month, the participants attended the program, enjoying the opportunity to spend time with others and to do interesting projects. By then it was apparent to the psychologist that her goal was inappropriate for the group of individuals she was treating and was in fact her goal, not theirs. As she came to know, understand, and respect these individuals, her programmatic goals shifted to emphasizing use of community resources to replicate the services of the day treatment center, where stays were limited. Instead of focusing on job skills, the psychologist worked to assist people in using public transportation, identifying inexpensive or free activities in the community, and establishing ties with community centers and churches. Eventually, a number of participants were successfully discharged to the community without recidivism to inpatient care. To an outsider, the intervention activities appeared unchanged, but to the psychologist and the clients, the goals had changed drastically.

Even such issues as who provides care must be considered thoughtfully. Particular sensitivity to gender concerns is often required. If it is unseemly in a particular culture for women to exercise, you may need to be creative about endurance training for mobility, perhaps having the person walk back and forth around the kitchen, where movement is considered acceptable, rather than between the parallel bars. Clinicians may well remember gender issues when intervention requires hands-on treatment, such as muscle massage. However, other interventions may also require sensitivity. A male client from a culture where masculine strength is highly valued may be reluctant to reveal personal problems to a female psychotherapist, for example.

Moreover, you must be prepared to abandon some of the goals you identify if they do not meet the needs of the individual. In describing the Lee family, Fadiman (1997) noted that they never felt it was essential that the child be seizure-free. Their world view accepted such seizures in a relatively matter-of-fact fashion. They would have been content to see the frequency and intensity reduced. The physicians, however, were determined to eliminate seizures altogether. Their goal led them to a number of interventions that were in conflict with the goals and values of the family.

Such conflicts can lead to ethical dilemmas for the practitioner when a particular treatment is perceived as essential and the individual or family reject it. Such dilemmas are discussed at greater length in Chapter 8; however, it is important to recognize the contribution of cultural beliefs to these situations. It is easy for us to conclude that we know what is best for our clients; however, such attitudes can be perceived as (and sometimes are) condescending and are ultimately counterproductive.

7-17. Reread the vignettes about Lia Lee that opened each chapter so far. Imagine yourself in each of the following roles:

Q

CULTURE AND HOSPICE CARE

Reese, Ahern, Nair, O'Faire, and Warren (1999) observed that African-American families tend to make little use of hospice services. Hospice is designed for individuals who are terminally ill. Its goals are to make the client comfortable physically during his or her last days, and to help the family and client deal effectively and supportively with the loss.

In African-American communities, according to Reese et al., it is generally believed that it is important to extend life as long as possible—a value in opposition to the beliefs of the hospice system. At the same time, in part because the church community is a major source of support in African-American communities, African-Americans may express greater acceptance of death than do other groups because of a belief that someone who dies is going to a "better place."

- The researchers were interested in knowing what they might do to encourage African-Americans to make more use of hospice. What kinds of information do you think they most need to collect? Based on what you know so far, how do you think they might have to adapt hospice care for this population?

- The public health nurse who had the opportunity to see Lia in her home context and did not consider her to be developmentally delayed
- The physician who reported the Lees to the authorities for their "neglect"
- Jeanine Hilt, the social worker
- Dee Korda, the foster mother
- The staff member who performed the spinal tap
- Lia's father, Nao Kao, or mother, Foua

Q 7-18. For each participant, state what you think may have been the primary motivating value for the person's behavior in the case. What cultural reinforcement is there in the typical American medical or health care setting for this value?

7-19. What do you consider the single most important question each participant could have asked to understand the situation better? What is the most important action each might have taken to help the Lee family deal with the situation? Who had the greatest responsibility for the terrible outcome for Lia?

Culturally Relevant Treatment Choice

A second factor in providing culturally sensitive intervention is the use of culturally relevant treatment. In rehabilitation, for example, it makes no sense to ask the individual to practice putting on pants if she never wears them. Careful assessment

and goal setting will help clarify the nature of the intervention. The client will almost certainly provide multiple clues to effective intervention during the assessment process.

The National Institute on Disability and Rehabilitation Research (1993) notes that

practitioners tend to view acculturation as a predictor of client success. If a client retains the language and continues to embrace the cultural characteristics of his or her home country, that client may be viewed by a rehabilitation counselor as being at high risk of not reaching rehabilitation goals.

Such beliefs on the part of practitioners must be carefully examined, as they suggest that goals have been determined by the clinician, not the client, or that the provider is responding to professional or organizational culture rather than approaching the situation in an independent and value-free fashion. It is more helpful to use information about culture and acculturation as a tool in identifying goals and intervention strategies rather than as a predictor of failure.

Consider, for example, a physical therapist working with an individual following a cerebrovascular accident. The therapist and the client may agree that mobility is an important issue and determine together that he will need to get around his home and the neighborhood. Therapists are well aware that they need to know about the home. How many steps? What kinds of floor surfaces? What kinds of doorways? Likewise, they need to know about the neighborhood. How far and under what circumstances does the client need to get around? Does he have a car? Will he ride the bus? Do his cultural values allow him to ask for help? Would an assistive device like a cane or walker be acceptable? However, it is of little value to facilitate walking with a walker if this is unacceptable to the individual in the context of his culture and community. Thought needs to be given to alternatives. If a cane is not an option, perhaps an umbrella or a walking stick is. Perhaps a circuitous route around the neighborhood will avoid uneven surfaces and minimize mobility difficulties.

A physician noting that a Muslim patient diagnosed with diabetes is not taking his medication needs to explore the reasons for this occurrence. A bit of probing and information-gathering may reveal that the Muslim religion requires avoidance of pork products, and that some forms of insulin are made from pigs. A change to a new form of insulin might solve the problem. If the physician is a woman, it may also help to ask a male colleague to convey instructions to the patient, as there may be rigid gender role definitions in Islamic cultures that might lead the patient to disregard a woman's recommendations.

An occupational therapist might find that cooking is a vital part of a woman's expected activities; the therapist needs to establish the kind of cooking and the circumstances under which it is done to ensure effective intervention. Practice making peanut butter and jelly sandwiches is not useful to someone whose primary diet is rice and stir-fried vegetables. Provision of adaptive equipment and alteration or modification of the activity must be approached with care, as both strategies may alter the activity beyond the person's recognition or acceptance. Following a cerebrovascular accident, making tortillas, typically a two-handed operation, may be difficult. The obvious solution of using a tortilla press may not be acceptable, so the therapist and client may need to work out a way to use the countertop and one hand to shape the dough. A weaver who can no longer manage complex patterns may not be satisfied by flat weaving, even though such weavings might have economic value.

A nurse may find a Chinese patient reluctant to accept pain medication following surgery. Such a patient might indicate that the pain is bearable and the medication unnecessary. The nurse may have read research journals indicating that recovery is aided by adequate pain control. She may discover that the patient is concerned about causing her unnecessary trouble when she has many other people for which to care. In this situation, the nurse may find it helpful to enlist the patient's help by noting that helping patients with their pain is her most important responsibility, and one on which she will be evaluated. Or, alternatively, she may decide that it is, after all, the patient's decision whether medication is warranted.

All of these situations require careful examination and exploration of alternatives. It is here that a focus on quality of life can be helpful. Perhaps a weaver can learn another type of creative activity, such as knitting, painting, or writing, or can find an alternative source of income. Perhaps a change in medication schedule will provide a better fit with a client's preferred lifestyle. Regardless of the recommended intervention strategy, it is vital to repeat it and regularly check its effectiveness, to maximize the likelihood that misunderstandings will be recognized and addressed.

It is possible that as clinicians expand their intercultural skills, they may find they can draw on knowledge of one group to assist another. For example, there is evidence that in some developing countries, many young people smoke, but most smoke only a few cigarettes a day and never move on to smoking more (Nichter, 2000). In addition, it has been documented that among new Hispanic immigrants to the United States, infant mortality is quite low in comparison to second-generation women or inner-city African-American women (James, 2000). In both cases, it is likely that cultural factors are responsible for these relatively positive outcomes and that identification of those cultural factors can inform interventions with Old American suburban young people, as well as with groups living in poverty.

7-20. Return to the case of Lia Lee. Think about the positive aspects of the Lees' parenting. What lessons might be drawn from their care of her? How might these lessons inform health care professionals about important emotional and psychological aspects of patient care?   **Q**

Care must be exercised in how a health provider conceptualizes intervention. A popular current perspective is that thoughtful intervention "empowers" the client (Kreps & Kunimoto, 1994). This notion suggests, however, that the clinician has the power and is willing to confer it on the client. In reality, both clinician and client bring power to the interaction, and the best interventions are those in which sharing of power is recognized and used strategically. It is easy to insert one's own views about the kinds of power that are desirable.

As we have mentioned previously, in Japan it is considered unacceptable to give people diagnoses of terminal illness for fear that they will become depressed and disheartened. Kreps and Kunimoto suggest that providing the diagnosis can be "empowering" because it allows the individual to make informed therapeutic decisions. Theirs is clearly a culture-bound assumption; it could be argued that "empowerment" is actually a different mechanism for imposing one's own power in the situation.

Of course, we do not mean that the clinician must never demonstrate superior knowledge or ability. In fact, certain kinds of healing depend on the client's faith in the healer's abilities. Among some Native Americans, for example, healing ceremonies are predicated on the healer's special knowledge and access to parts of the world set off from everyday life. In clinical encounters, likewise, it is often helpful to convey the presence of special knowledge. However, this process is different from insistence that one is right. Traditional healers make their expertise known but wait to be invited to employ it.

A final step in providing culturally relevant care is the evaluation of outcomes. Evaluation is essential not only to the assessment of a current case, but in order to create a knowledge base for future reference. Because each situation is unique, it is only through careful reflection that health care providers can determine what strategies might be tried again. Chapter 8 considers the evaluation process in detail.

✎ NOTES ✐

✎ NOTES ✎

8

Assessing Intercultural Interactions and Interventions

CHAPTER OBJECTIVES

By the end of this chapter, the reader will be able to:

1. Discuss the impact of cultural factors on ethical dilemmas and decisions.
2. Define five tiers for ethical decision-making.
3. Describe strategies for approaching ethical dilemmas.
4. Define the characteristics of successful cultural encounters.
5. Identify mechanisms for assessing cultural variables in clinical encounters.
6. Describe the use of triangulation to assess effectiveness, including the use of videotaping, case discussions, neutral observers, treatment team interaction, and client feedback.
7. Describe the process of meta-ethnography as a mechanism for evaluating clinical effectiveness.
8. List and describe five elements of culturally inclusive therapy.

THE STORY OF LIA LEE

After removing Lia from the hospital against medical advice, the Lees provided her with constant attention and care that they were convinced was preferable to the unsuccessful medical interventions. They fed her by dripping food, sometimes prechewed by her mother, down her throat in small amounts. They bathed her with herbal infusions and massaged her, keeping her clean and neat. A home health nurse visited, and instructed them how to take a pulse, looking at a watch to count seconds. The Lees had no watch and could not recognize numbers. The nurse also advised prune juice for constipation caused by Lia's lack of movement, writing the word PRUNE in large letters on a piece of paper to be sure they understood. The Lees did not know what prune juice was and could not read the word. Jeanine Hilt, the social worker who had followed the case for some time, worked the system to get the Lees a hospital bed for Lia. Lia never used the bed, since she slept each night with her parents in a small room cramped by the unused hospital bed.

Lia is now a comatose but attractive, clean, and well-groomed child, attended to by parents who are now classified as exemplary, rather than as difficult, slow, and noncompliant. The Lees were right that the hospital made Lia sicker. On the other hand, if she had still been in Laos, Lia would probably have died in infancy. "American medicine had both preserved her life and compromised it" (Fadiman, 1997, p. 258).

After the fact, both the professionals and the Lees continued to examine the process that had led to such a dismal outcome for Lia. The Lees expressed considerable sympathy for "Lia's doctors." They recognized that the physicians and other staff had tried to help her, although they continued to maintain that medical care had been unsuccessful. The physicians agreed with this assessment and were deeply troubled by it. They had put tremendous effort into trying to help a patient they perceived as very difficult and a family whom they had originally found unsympathetic. They knew that they had made multiple errors in judgment, in part because of their failure to address adequately the cultural factors that were so prominent in the situation.

According to Kleinman (1980), several specific strategies might have altered the outcome.

First, get rid of the term 'compliance.' It's a lousy term. It implies moral hegemony.... Second, instead of looking at a model of coercion, look at a model of mediation.... Decide what's critical and be willing to compromise on everything else. Third, you need to understand that as powerful an influence as the culture of the Hmong patient and her family is in this case, the culture of biomedicine is equally powerful. If you can't see that your own culture has its own set of interests, emotions, and biases, how can you expect to deal successfully with someone else's culture? (p. 261)

Summarized from Fadiman, A. (1997). *The spirit catches you and you fall down.* New York: Noonday Press.

INTRODUCTION

Our goal in writing this book was to make the cultural component of therapeutic practices explicit and responsive to theory. We wish to transform good practice from common sense and professional tradition to a more informed practice—to make certain unconscious facets of therapy practice conscious by focusing on culture (Hahn, 1995).

In previous chapters we discussed culture emergent, how it affects behavior, how to use ethnographic methods to recognize cultural differences, how to negotiate cultural differences in working with clients, and how to evaluate clients and design interventions in a diverse world through a process of mutual cultural accommodation. In this chapter we offer an approach to therapist–client interactions that takes cultural differences into account.

We begin with a consideration of ethics in intercultural situations. The approach we take toward ethics in health care differs from that of most philosophers. Rather than search for universal ethical principles, ethnographers are more likely to situate the moral dimensions of health care in local ethical practices, thus emphasizing social practices rather than abstract moral propositions (Marshall & Koenig, 1996). There are complex relationships between health care providers and their clients, among clinicians and various health professionals, and between clinicians and the larger society. All of

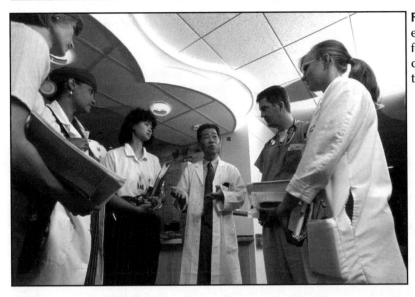

Figure 8-1. Case conferences offer opportunities for individuals of different cultures to share perspectives and information.

these relationships influence daily decision-making, and each type of relationship carries ethical implications. When a therapist does not share the same cultural values and assumptions about ethical behavior with a client, the implications can be significant (Figure 8-1).

After exploring the ethical parameters of practitioner–client interaction, we next summarize methods for assessing and improving the success of interactions and interventions in intercultural situations. We suggest principles of good practice that will maximize beneficial treatment outcomes while preserving the ideal of professional ethics.

Finally, we close with a summary statement of five elements of **culturally inclusive** health care. These are elements you must recognize, believe, and put into practice if you are to be a culturally inclusive practitioner.

A CONSIDERATION OF ETHICS

Ethics are about doing what is right. Behaving ethically assumes you know what is right and what is wrong. Some ethical choices are relatively simple: it is wrong to kill another person, it is right to take care of your family. What if these two are in conflict, however? Suppose an intruder threatens your loved ones. Is it all right in those circumstances to kill another human being? For many of us it is difficult to know with certainty what is right all the time and in all situations. All too often we are confronted with decisions that cannot be categorized as absolutely, positively, beyond a shadow of a doubt, totally and completely right or wrong.

Health care ethics are culturally constructed. They reflect a tradition of beliefs and a set of preferred behaviors about health, sickness, and health care practices. As Marshall and Koenig (1996) state

[T]he purview of medical ethics across cultures includes the lived experience of human suffering in the context of disease, the moral discourse of healers and patients, the development and use of healing modalities, the professional organization of practitioners, and the social and economic regulation of medical environments. (pp. 350–351)

Although ethics may seem abstract, having little to do with real life, you carry out ethical decision-making every day. A clear understanding of ethics emphasizes social practices (i.e., the experiences and interactions of health care workers, clients, and families in everyday life) rather than abstract moral propositions. Ethics should not be divorced from clients' suffering or the hopes and fears of their families.

The practical question with regard to the study of ethics is how cognitively aware you are of those decisions. What follows is a review of some considerations that may help you evaluate your individual responsibilities within broad ethical parameters.

The Role of Authority in Ethical Decision-Making

The role of authority in ethical decision-making is basic to determining right actions. To illustrate, consider the examples of two contrasting positions: the authoritarian and situational approaches to ethical decisions. The authoritarian approach assumes that when we make choices about what to do, we can rely on a normative standard within society as a whole. Generally, authoritarians believe that there is a single right behavior for any situation. The standard may be a list of specific rules for each circumstance one might encounter—for example, religious tenets—or a set of civil laws or professional principles that can be used in making decisions.

This normative standard upon which ethical choices are made is derived from an authority higher than the individual. The authority may be a supernatural one, as interpreted by religious specialists such as priests or ministers. The authority may be derived from a representative council chosen for their wisdom and experience. For example, there are ethics committees for many professions to determine correct and proper professional behavior for members.

The situational approach assumes that there is no authority outside the individual that can provide a set of principles for determining right behavior in all circumstances. Although situationalists may believe that an individual should consider traditional wisdom collected over the generations, the responsibility for making ethically sound decisions rests squarely with the individual. Situationalists accept the burden of not always being able to know with certainty the right course. Indeed, they would argue that accepting this uncertainty is an essential ingredient for responsible behavior.

Q

8-1. Think about the difference between authoritarian and situational approaches to ethics. High-profile cases offer opportunities to explore our ethical approaches and analyze our discomfort with them. With a partner, choose one of the three examples given below and discuss it, keeping clear, independent notes about your and your partner's ethical positions on the case.

- An adult woman, 5 1/2 months pregnant, is in an automobile accident that leaves her brain dead but the fetus uninjured. Mechanical devices can keep her body systems functioning long enough for the fetus to come to term and be born alive and healthy. Her husband does not want to keep his wife alive in this way, but the woman's parents are anxious to have a grandchild. What do you think should happen?
- An elderly man, widowed and suffering from lung cancer and heart disease, has a stroke with resultant hemiplegia. In addition, he experiences a great deal of pain. The doctor is reluctant to recommend therapy, because it will increase the man's pain and his cancer is expected to progress rapidly. The family wants the man to have aggressive therapy. The man has some aphasia and is having difficulty expressing his own views. What do you think should be done?
- A young couple discover that they are infertile and decide to have artificial insemination with donor sperm and the woman's egg. The embryo is then implanted in a surrogate mother's womb. Amniocentesis reveals that the fetus suffers from a genetic disease and will be born severely retarded and physically abnormal. The couple wants the child and the surrogate wants to abort it. What do you think?

8-2. Once you have concluded your discussion, evaluate your decision-making strategies as either authoritarian or situational. If authoritarian, what standard principles or rules were used to guide your thinking? If situational, what were the most significant factors in the situation for the position you took?

8-3. Imagine that you are involved somehow in the chosen case in your professional role. Assume that your own position is not the one selected by the parties to the situation. What difficulties do you expect to have in accepting and adjusting to what you think is an unethical outcome?

Ethics and Health Issues

In health care, there are ethical decisions to be made concerning issues such as birth control, sexually transmitted diseases, the use of technology to reverse infertility, do-not-resuscitate orders, allocation of donated organs, triage decisions, distribution of health care resources, assisted suicide, abortion, and false reporting on records that allows patients necessary treatment when the patient cannot afford it, among many other examples. Moreover, there are new dimensions of science and technology that entail ethical considerations, such as genetic engineering and the cloning of human beings. It is expected that in the next few years cloning technology will make it possible to grow partial human

THE ROLE OF AUTHORITY IN DECISION-MAKING: AUTHORITARIAN VS. SITUATIONAL VIEWS

Authoritarian:

- Ethics must be grounded in collective wisdom.
- Most individuals are not sufficiently wise to make ethical determinations on their own.
- Most individuals are not sufficiently strong to do what is right—they must submit to social sanctions to guide them to right decisions.
- There is one right way. When two principles seem to conflict, the conflict is only apparent because the law or other authority also prioritizes these principles, so you can always determine what is right.
- Such conflicts are best decided through interpretation (usually by wise men).

Situational:

- Individuals should consider collective wisdom as a source for ethical decision-making.
- Although individuals are not equally wise, each must assume responsibility for his or her actions.
- Social sanctions are useful to provide for social order, but an ethical individual may choose to violate those guides.
- Individuals must decide what is the right course and then accept responsibility for their own actions.
- Frequently, principles are in conflict and decisions must be made *in situ*, not *a priori*.

fetuses to harvest organs for transplants. Then, all of us will have to confront serious ethical questions. What are the ethical implications of these examples of biomedical technology? What can be done to limit unethical outcomes? Difficult cases already abound. How would you respond to the ones presented in the "Difficult Cases" box on page 160?

Determining Right in a Diverse Society

Doing what is right can create special problems in pluralistic societies marked by a diversity of religious and moral traditions. Such diversity can create situations where the right behavior of one group is in conflict with the right behavior of another.

The golden rule of civil society is that your individual freedom is possible only if you allow others their freedom. Of course, even this rule assumes the presence of sufficient agreement among society's constituencies to maintain minimal social structures and contracts (i.e., an agreement on how society generally ought to work).

Moreover, the rule of the majority cannot be assumed as a moral imperative. The fact that those with great power or those with the support of a majority of voters decide on a course of action or a particular law does not mean that action or that law is morally right. For example, in the United States the right of women to vote began as a minority movement attacking the position of the majority. Although it took decades to change existing statutes, few today would question that denying women the right to vote would be an immoral position. In other countries, however, the disenfranchisement of women is still the norm.

Similarly, in many countries health care is considered a right, and health care payment is provided for every citizen. In the United States, however, attempts to provide some sort of universal health insurance have met with resistance, and a significant portion of the population does not have insurance to cover health care costs.

Both of these examples underscore the fact that ethics are grounded in time and culture; they cannot be divorced from a given historical moment nor from a specific cultural context. Ethics, including health care ethics, "are culturally constituted, embedded in religious and political ideologies that influence individuals and communities at particular

DIFFICULT CASES: WHAT DO YOU THINK?

- Some states have laws that require physicians to report the names of people who test positive for HIV, the virus that causes AIDS, and to notify their sex partners. Critics of HIV notification legislation believe that mandatory reporting will deter some people from seeking testing and treatment. What do you think?

- A young man is brought into the emergency room following an automobile accident. He is found to be brain dead. His father asks that sperm be obtained so that at a later time his fianceé can be inseminated (Nolan, 1998). Some ethicists question whether it is right to deliberately bring a child into the world with a dead father and if it is appropriate to perform a medical procedure to assuage the grief of a surviving family member. Others have stated that this procedure raises questions about reproductive freedom and men giving their consent to be fathers. What do you think?

- A 75-year-old retired widow has become increasingly physically and cognitively impaired over the last 3 years. Following discharge from a hospital stay necessitated by the woman's inability to manage the medications she needs to control her congestive heart failure, the insurance company is uncertain about whether to pay for home health care although the woman expresses a strong wish to return home. The company fears that she may be at risk if supported in returning home rather than to a nursing home (Crigger, 1998). Some ethicists would argue that individuals with cognitive impairments have the same right to self-determination as other individuals. Others have argued that special protection is needed for such individuals. What is your view of this dilemma?

- The parents of an 11-year-old developmentally disabled girl want to have her surgically sterilized because they believe that her limited intellectual capacity would not permit her to make responsible contraceptive choices nor to be an adequate parent if she became pregnant (Crigger, 1998). Do loving and concerned parents have the right to make this kind of decision for their child?

- A physician on a rehabilitation unit is working with an 85-year-old man who has just had surgery for a hip fracture. The man, now 24 hours post-surgery, has an extremely low blood count as a result of the fracture and subsequent surgery. Because of his low blood count, it is not safe for him to stand, meaning that he cannot begin a rehabilitation program. However, reimbursement rules state that rehabilitation must begin within 48 hours of admission to the unit. Thus, the physician feels he must either provide a blood transfusion, which is very frightening to the man, or discharge him. There is no time to arrange a nursing home stay, and the man broke his hip while traveling in a city where he knows no one. Is the physician right to insist on a transfusion? Can the nurses and therapists help him find another solution?

biographical and historical moments" (Marshall & Koenig, 1996, p. 357). However, as societies evolve, so do ethical behaviors.

When political power is equated with moral right there is the danger of ignoring individual rights and needs. This danger may be seen with regard to women's rights and gender equity, rights regardless of sexual orientation, the right to control one's reproductive potential, the right to define life, the right to end a life, and even the right to equitable health care. In all of these cases the rights of a single societal constituency or political elite in society may be pitted against those of other individuals.

The question of power is a central one in health care ethics. Divergent beliefs about the exercise of power and control in a therapeutic relationship have an impact on clinician–client interactions, as well as on the outcomes of treatment. There is also a tension between a clinician's power to influence health care decisions and a client's ability and desire to exercise choice in decision-making.

Clients and their families are especially vulnerable when they are seeking health care. As Marshall (1992) notes, they may be struggling to make sense of a moral world gone awry. They may feel that they are central characters in *When Bad Things Happen to Good People* (Kushner, 1992). At such times, the position of the clinician may lead the client to perceive that the health care provider is one who speaks with moral authority, and the client may accede some of her or his own autonomy to the clinician.

A Draft for an Ethics of Health Care in Five Tiers

How does the clinician deal with a situation in which the client's cultural values are perceived as interfering with the clinician's perceived good outcomes (e.g., refusal of treatment, treatment directed toward goals that conflict with the client's cultural system)? For example, how can a clinician deal with a Jehovah's Witness family that is refusing a potentially life-saving transfusion for their child?

Raymond A. Belliotti (1993) has provided a balanced consideration of sexual ethics, which we have adapted for presentation here as a tentative statement on ethics of health care. This statement is presented for purposes of reflection and discussion. Note that in Belliotti's five-tiered framework, Tier 1 is primary; only if the act passes evaluation at this level does one need to consider subsequent tiers.

Tier 1: Libertarian Agreement. The parties (i.e., the clinician and the client or the client's guardian), possessing the basic capacities necessary for autonomous choice, must agree to a particular intervention, or decision not to act, without force, fraud, or explicit duress.

Tier 2: General Moral Considerations. Decisions about health care are not different from other types of moral decision-making. Some basic principles, including the consideration of motives and intentions, must apply. The general moral principles acknowledged in most societies include the following: keep promises, tell the truth, return favors, aid others in distress, make reparation for harm to others that is one's own fault, oppose injustices, promote just institutions, assume one's fair share of societal burdens, avoid causing pain or suffering to others, avoid inexcusable killing of others, and avoid stealing or otherwise depriving others of their property.

Tier 3: Exploitation. Any exploitative or coercive act is morally impermissible, even if the exploitation or coercion is subtle. Exploitation occurs when one party (e.g., the clinician) takes advantage of another party's (e.g., the client's) attributes or situation to exact personal gain or gain for the exploiter's compatriots (e.g., a clinic or hospital).

Tier 4: Third Party Effects. When the considered health care activity meets the previous ethical considerations, it may still be morally impermissible if anyone not directly involved in the act will nevertheless be harmed as a result (e.g., a spouse or child might suffer indirectly as a result of health care behaviors).

Tier 5: Wider Social Context. Even if a health care action meets all other criteria, it might be morally impermissible if it reinforces oppressive social roles, contributes to continued social inequality, gives rise to new forms of oppression, or otherwise adds to the contamination of the wider social and political context surrounding health care.

Q

8-4. Before reading further, think carefully about these proposed ethical guidelines. Are they more authoritarian, more situational, or neutral in approach? Using the case you and a partner considered in exercises 8-1 through 8-3, work through the tiers as a guide to reaching an ethical outcome. What problems do you encounter? How well do the guidelines cover your case?

8-5. Consider Tier 2. Which of the following phrases carries culturally defined assumptions? What effect does the existence of these assumptions have on the likely universality of the principles?
- Tell the truth
- Make reparation for harm
- Oppose injustice
- Just institutions
- Stealing
- One's fair share
- Avoid causing pain
- Inexcusable killing

Note that Tier 1 in the above model assumes individual autonomy is good and desirable. This assumption is common in Western societies, especially in the United States, where there is a strong cultural bias toward individualism. Traditional Western health care ethics presume "an individuated self, set apart from the collective experience of family or community" (Marshall & Koenig, 1996, p. 356). This pattern is not the norm in many cultures where health care decisions are deferred to the family, the oldest relative, a community council, or a religious leader.

To date, ethicists largely have ignored cultural differences, despite the fact that encounters between clinicians and clients with different cultures have become routine (Marshall & Koenig, 1996, p. 367). Given that many of the world's societies have become pluralistic, it is likely that we will see more studies that focus on these issues in the future. In the meantime, each individual provider

CHILD ABUSE?

A nurse in the emergency room notices that the child she is treating has multiple bruises on the chest and arms. The nurse knows that multiple bruises may be a sign of child abuse and that she is bound both by law and by ethical principles to report her suspicions. However, the nurse also notes that the child's family is first-generation Vietnamese. She is familiar with the custom of coin-rubbing as a healing strategy in Vietnamese culture and knows that it often leaves bruises. She finds no other signs of abuse.

- What are the nurse's options, based on the law?
- How can the nurse deal with the situation in a culturally sensitive way?

must make decisions based on reflection and a consideration of the available information.

Doing What Is Right

You are the only one who can decide what is the right action for you, although others—professional ethics boards and their guidelines, legislators and legal professionals, your supervisor, the client's family—may determine what action you actually take in certain contexts. If you are more cognitively oriented in your decision-making style, you may carefully think everything through. If you are more intuitively guided in your decision-making strategies, you may rely on your instincts. The reality is that the two are interactive in all of us. Whether you think you are being rational or emotional, you are undoubtedly acting in response to the value orientations and accumulated past experiences that you have acquired through education and socialization.

Ethicists seldom agree on absolutes. However, the following basic ethical considerations may be a foundation for your decisions about health and health care.

- Do nothing to harm another, physically or psychologically. This restriction applies to third party and indirect effects your behavior will have on others. The group of affected others includes potential others, such as future offspring.

- Never use force or coercion. This blanket statement refers to psychological pressure as well as physical force. Do not exploit the weakness or subordinate status (e.g., social, political, educational, or cultural) of others, and do not try to persuade someone to do something he or she does not want to do.

- Take responsibility for your actions. Use no deception and break no promises. Make it clear what you intend to do and why.

8-6. Carefully consider these distilled guidelines. How well do they conform to your own decision-making in the case you studied in exercises 8-1 through 8-3? Do you think they are an improvement over the five tiers approach you applied to that case? How so, or why not? Can you identify problems, difficulties, unaddressed issues in their application to that case?

8-7. Reread the vignette about Lia Lee that opened this chapter. How might the situation have been different if all the health care providers involved—emergency room person-

GIFTS AS AN ETHICAL DILEMMA

In some Jewish and Korean traditions, gift-giving to care providers is an important mechanism for establishing reciprocity in the relationship. It is not unusual for clients or their families to give a gift of money. It is also not unusual for health care organizations to have policies that prohibit staff from accepting money from patients.

- What is the clinician's responsibility in this situation?
- How can such a situation be handled in a culturally sensitive and ethical manner?

nel, the home health care nurse, the social worker, the physicians, the technicians—had used these guidelines to govern their behavior?

Q 8-8. What ethical guidelines do you think Lia's parents were using as the situation unfolded?

Postponing the consideration of ethics until the moment of crisis does not relieve you of the responsibility of your choices. Nor does accepting the suggestions of another or giving in to pressure relieve you of the responsibility of your actions. Moreover, when it comes to ethics, doing nothing (i.e., taking no purposive action) is doing something. There simply is no way to avoid responsibility for your behavior.

ASSESSING INTERACTION AND INTERVENTION

With an awareness of some of the potential difficulties for the clinician and the client in intercultural situations, we are ready to consider guidelines for negotiating interactions and interventions in such settings. We want to make clear that the general approach is the same for all clients. As we have stressed previously, the possibility of **intracultural variability** is always present. As a therapist you do not necessarily have obvious clues (e.g., language, physical appearance, clothing) that will alert you to the likelihood of cultural variation. However, once you have become aware that substantial cultural variation between you and your client may exist, you should be especially sensitive in interactions with that client.

Successful Clinician–Client Interactions

The goal for the clinician is the same for all clients: to facilitate the clients' wishes and help them move toward the achievement of their own goals. Clients' wishes are grounded in their life experiences, and understanding these experiences and related values and beliefs is critical to the success of intervention. The health care provider can offer specific knowledge and skills to clients, helping them match their wishes to the realities of the situation.

In Chapters 5 through 7, we discussed strategies that can be helpful in addressing cultural issues in intervention. However, the health care encounter is not complete until its effectiveness has been addressed. In order to determine success, it is vital to recognize the characteristics of successful intercultural encounters.

One strategy that is sometimes recommended is self-assessment of the therapist using one of the many published instruments that emphasize cultural competency. Among the instruments available are the *Intercultural Development Inventory* (Hammer, 1998); the *Multicultural Counseling Inventory* (Sodowsky, Taffe, Gutkin, & Wise, 1994); and the *Inventory to Assess the Process of Cultural Competence Among Health Care Professionals* (Camphina-Bacote, 1999). Allotey, Nikles, and Manderson (1998) have developed a series of checklists that enable clinicians to monitor the process as it proceeds. They offer lists that examine communication effectiveness, use of interpreters, staff attitudes toward cultural diversity, assessment of culture, cultural formulation, and so on. Another instrument, the *Multicultural Sensitivity Scale* (Jibaja, Sebastian, Kingery, & Holcomb, 2000) includes items like these (p. 81):

- "When I observe the hardships of some people, I understand why they are not proud of their ethnic identity...."
- "I prefer working with people with whom I can identify ethnically...."
- "I would feel more relaxed if I could work with people of my own ethnic group."

The respondent rates each item on a scale from 1 (strongly disagree) to 6 (strongly agree). Assuming that the respondent answers accurately and has sufficient insight to know what answers are accurate, these kinds of instruments may provide some general information about attitudes about culture. However, these are major assumptions that may not be true. Even if the assumptions are met and the scores reflect some kind of general measure of attitude, they say nothing about how those attitudes are translated into action, nor about the degree of success with which the actions are received. Thus, standardized instruments are not a useful strategy for determining the success of evaluation and intervention strategies in intercultural contexts. Our emphasis is on behavior and actions. We stress attitude—what we call the ethnographic mindset—primarily as a way of orienting our awareness so that information can reach us and guide our behavior.

Successful Evaluations

A successful evaluation is one that identifies client problems from the perspective of the individual. Cultural factors are addressed explicitly, as are social and environmental factors. Such information permits establishment of goals that are consistent with the client's beliefs and are valued and meaningful to the individual. In both evaluation and treatment planning, cultural factors will be clearly addressed, demonstrating real concern for the individual rather than *pro forma* selection of goals. The assessment provides sufficient information that the intervention plan can be recognized as having been developed by a particular clinician working with a unique patient.

Given current constraints in the health care environment, successful evaluations are efficient and establish goals for which the facility will receive payment. It is unreasonable and unrealistic to assume that clinicians can ignore these constraints. We have provided some strategies for accomplishing this kind of evaluation and address (below) the means by which success can be evaluated.

Whereas successful evaluation and treatment planning respect the clients' wishes and are respectful of their culture, it is not required that clinicians abandon their own values and beliefs. Treatment is a process of negotiation, in which each individual has a right to feel respected. One therapist, for example, told the story of her interaction with a young man with a new spinal cord injury. His occupation prior to his injury had been dealing drugs, to which he wanted to return. The therapist disapproved of this career. The client and the therapist had to engage in serious discussion to reach an acceptable compromise, one in which they agreed to address functional goals without regard to the work to which he might return.

In addition, clinicians must give consideration to situations in which the client cannot make the decision (e.g., in the case of a very young child or someone with a severe cognitive impairment or who is from a culture in which someone other than the client is the primary decision-maker). Such cases involve additional complexity, because the clinician must obtain and weigh information from multiple sources in considering intervention.

Q 8-9. The staff involved with Lia Lee's case attempted evaluation, as described in the vignette in this chapter. How do you view the way in which goals were set, treatment plans determined, and outcomes assessed? How might the providers have used regular, ongoing evaluation as a strategy to improve care during this case?

Successful Interventions

Successful interventions are those that enable clients to reach the goals that have been negotiated in the assessment and planning process. Ideally, these interventions allow clients to return to meaningful life in the environments from which they have come. When that outcome is not possible, they allow clients to determine what alternatives will be satisfying to them and facilitate their entry into the new environment.

The role of the health care provider may be the same with all clients, but clients with substantial cultural variation may require flexibility and adaptability on the part of the clinician. The clinician may need to serve as broker or facilitator as information about cultural issues becomes clear. It is neither expected nor possible for the clinician to have complete and entirely accurate information about the client's multiple cultural affiliations, but it is essential that the clinician recognize the possibility of conflicting vantages and the need for mutual cultural accommodation.

IMPROVING SERVICE IN INTERCULTURAL SITUATIONS

The perspective of culture emergent establishes that each clinician and each client is a unique individual whose cultural beliefs and values are expressed from the specific individual vantage that reflects personal experience and the **interactional moment**. For this reason, it is impossible to know all there is to know about culture or to apply a set of rules that will ensure successful intervention. However, careful examination of outcomes of each encounter can yield important information that can improve future interventions.

Clinicians who work in environments where there are significant numbers of intercultural encounters with clients may institute procedures designed specifically to improve outcomes for those clients. Such procedures can be especially helpful for providers who have little awareness of culture and how it affects therapy or little knowledge of the cultural beliefs and behaviors of those clients.

Just as ethnographic methods can facilitate effective cross-cultural communication and intervention, qualitative research methods can facilitate evaluation of those interactions. Interactions can be thought of as data to be analyzed, and methods that ensure qualitative rigor can effectively guide analysis of therapeutic situations. In examining data,

YOU CANNOT ALWAYS GET IT RIGHT

His Holiness, the spiritual leader of an Indian Orthodox Christian Church, became a patient in an American hospital when he fell ill during a visit to the American Diocese. His condition required cardiac catheterization and open heart surgery. Because it was determined that, despite the extraordinary precautions taken, his body had become contaminated during the procedure, there was a 10-day delay during which he had to undergo a purification ceremony before he could have open heart surgery.

How had he become contaminated? First of all, the surgical team members had allowed non-Orthodox Christians [to] do the electrocardiogram and blood withdrawal and to shave the groin on His Holiness. Priests and bishops within this church must avoid exposing their bodies to any female in order to maintain purity. Although there were no female members caring directly for His Holiness, the director of the catheterization laboratory was a female. Even though she was in the back room operating the x-ray machines, this was a breach of sexual segregation: His Holiness' private parts had been exposed to a woman.

Although he had not received any food prior to surgery—as is common when anesthesia is used—the medical team allowed him to receive holy communion the morning of his heart catheterization. Unfortunately, this led to a cardinal sin. After surgery, His Holiness vomited and the medical team discarded the emesis. Holy communion is the blood and body of Jesus Christ; when he vomited the communion, His Holiness was in essence vomiting Christ. The hospital staff should have saved the emesis to be drunk by the priests and bishops there to take care of His Holiness. Drinking the emesis is considered a very holy act and will wash away one's sins.

From Galanti, G. (1997). *Caring for patients from different cultures: Case studies from American hospitals* (2nd ed., p. 41). Philadelphia: University of Pennsylvania Press. © 1997 Geri-Ann Galanti. Reprinted with permission from the University of Pennsylvania Press.

- How many Indian Orthodox Christian spiritual leaders have you known? How much have you read about the beliefs and practices of such individuals?
- How could you learn about the values and behaviors of such individuals?
- Under what circumstances should it occur to you to ask about practices concerning disposal or use of emesis from spiritual leaders?

That last question was a trick. You will never think to ask for such information and will never be able to avoid every cultural mis-step. You might reasonably think to discuss in detail issues about gender of care providers, because this kind of concern is found in many cultures. You will not find very many examples in which emesis is the center of focus. The best you can do is to get as much information as possible in each situation, act as thoughtfully as possible with the information you have obtained, and be prepared to apologize or otherwise make amends when you encounter a problem.

qualitative researchers are concerned with **trustworthiness** (i.e., the dependability, credibility, transferability, and applicability of the information gathered). Providers are concerned with dependability because they want to know that their information is reliable. They are concerned with the credibility, or believability, of the data. Transferability is important because the ultimate goal of intervention is to make a difference to the individual in situations outside the clinical encounter. Because each intercultural encounter is in some sense unique, applicability may be of somewhat less concern, as it can be assumed that data will not transfer perfectly to another situation. However, at least some of the information gleaned from one client is likely to apply to others, and reflection on one encounter should illuminate others. Recall the case described in an earlier chapter of the hearing-impaired client who was told that he had tested positive for HIV; he was pleased to learn that the test was positive because of the usual meaning of the word "positive."

Q

8-10. What might the nurse have learned from this encounter?

8-11. How might she apply that new information in future situations?

The most helpful mechanisms for ensuring trustworthiness of the information are those that provide additional vantages for the clinician. One such strategy is **triangulation** (Bechtel, Davidhizar, & Bunting, 2000), a mechanism by which various information sources are checked against each other. Among the strategies for triangulation are: 1) data triangulation, in which various forms of data (e.g., standardized instruments, assessment data) are checked for consistency; 2) investigator triangulation, in which two individuals check their observations during debriefing or other conversation; and 3) interdisciplinary triangulation, involving comparison of perspectives of various professionals from differing disciplines. In clinical situations, triangulation can be useful in confirming interpretations of evaluation information, as well as the value of goals and intervention strategies. **Member checking** is a particular form of triangulation in which the "other" data source is the client him- or herself (Krefting, 1991). Asking the client to reflect on your inferences can yield valuable insights about the usefulness of your intervention.

Value of the "Treatment Team" Approach

One useful strategy for examining outcomes is discussion in a treatment team. This form of triangulation represents a mechanism for peer debriefing. We have discussed the fact that each profession has its own culture, and its culture is enacted in choices that professionals make in their interventions. Often, hearing from someone whose perspective differs from yours can provide valuable insight into your own beliefs and how they affect your treatment choices.

Consider this example, which was recently reported to us. An elderly African-American woman was being treated in an outpatient rehabilitation clinic of a large hospital for consequences of a cardiovascular accident. Typically, her daughter brought her to her treatment sessions and waited while she was seen. After the first two visits, the physical therapist approached the patient, only to have her daughter shout, "You aren't touching her. You hurt her. You don't understand our culture—

only *she* can treat her." She pointed to an African-American occupational therapist who also worked in the clinic. The therapist acceded to the request to avoid further confrontation, but the situation became the topic of careful analysis in the next treatment team meeting.

As we mentioned earlier, situations may not always concern the most obvious cultural differences such as ethnicity or national origin, although these categories may at first obscure our view of the more subtle sources. In this case, as the Old American physical therapist and the African-American occupational therapist discussed the situation, it became clear that, in fact, the problem did not relate to a cultural gap between African-Americans and Old Americans. Rather, it related to differences between the professional cultures of physical therapy, in which pain is sometimes a necessary consequence of treatment, and occupational therapy, which is more likely to emphasize processing of emotional reactions and in which pain is less likely to occur during treatment.

In this example, it was the cross-disciplinary discussion between therapists perceiving the situation from different professional as well as other cultural vantages that facilitated understanding of the problem. In the next treatment session, the occupational therapist was able to reintroduce the physical therapist, inaugurate a discussion of concerns about physical therapy treatment, and help negotiate a resolution in which the physical therapist did not push quite as hard; the woman and her daughter came to recognize the need for a certain amount of pain.

8-12. On hearing about this example, one physical therapist we know became somewhat disturbed and asked, "Why would you say that physical therapists always cause pain and occupational therapists never do?" Reread the example above. Does it say that physical therapists always cause pain and occupational therapists never do?

Q

8-13. Why do you think the physical therapist might have reacted as she did? How might her reaction relate to her vantage?

8-14. In your work or study setting, do you have the possibility of working in cross-professional teams? What advantages and disadvantages have you observed, heard about, or can you imagine for working in such teams?

Case Discussions

In addition to team meetings about existing situations and cases, it can be helpful to have regular case discussions about real or simulated cases. Care providers who have been in a setting for a while may have information from the vantage of greater experience that can identify typical kinds of cultural misunderstandings that seem frequent in that setting. Likewise, they may have acquired specific wisdom about solutions to those misunderstandings or strategies for avoiding them altogether. At the same time, newer providers may have learned information in their training that can refresh the perspective of the more experienced providers. In addition, they may be able to recognize stereotypes that longer-term staff have developed that are counterproductive and assist them in reframing their observations.

Use of Neutral Observers

It should be clear by now that confidence in the idea of a "neutral" observer is somewhat misplaced. No observing mind is ever completely without assumptions and vantage. However, it is possible to find people who do not have direct, immediate, emotional responses to a situation, whose vantage is somewhat more objective. The actors in a health care situation always have some degree of investment in it. Clients are anxious to please the clinician, eager for a "cure" or a return to pre-difficulty functioning. They may feel frustrated, frightened, or powerless. Providers want to feel that what they are doing is of value and is appreciated by their client. They also want to feel that they are doing a good job as defined by their profession and the facility in which they work. These varying emotional needs may be in conflict and can affect the ability of the participants in the encounter to process events.

In the case of Lia Lee, for example, the Lees were focused exclusively on Lia and were worried and anxious. They perceived the staff as mysterious, powerful, and frightening. The staff were also worried and anxious. Like the Lees, they wanted Lia to get better. They perceived the Lees as intransigent and difficult, and they dreaded seeing them arrive in the emergency room. During the writing of her book, Fadiman (1997), a "neutral" observer, was able to explore the emotions of the participants around the difficult encounter and come to a more comfortable understanding, recognizing that both were doing the best that was possible given their understanding of the case. Had Fadiman, or someone like her, appeared earlier, it is possible that the outcome of the case would have been better. This possibility points to the need for therapists to consider obtaining outside views and to process their observations with knowledgeable individuals not directly involved in specific clinical situations.

The Use of Video to Study Yourself, Client, and Others

Videotaping is another form of triangulation, used in many training environments to enhance insight and interpersonal skills. Often by seeing ourselves from the outside, we can learn a great deal about our behavior. For reasons of privacy and confidentiality, it is not possible to tape every, or even most, encounters. However, occasional taping can be a valuable mechanism for assessing intercultural competence. Such tapes can be used as a means of stimulating discussion in team meetings or training sessions. Permission must be obtained from the client, but many are willing to agree if they understand the purpose of the tape. Some clients also benefit from seeing the tapes, which can be used not only for training the professional, but as a feedback mechanism for clients who might otherwise not be aware of their status or, in the case of longitudinal taping, the therapeutic progress, which becomes evident while watching tapes. Clinicians can include language in preliminary information to clients that includes a request for permission to tape interactions for the specific purpose of quality improvement.

Client Feedback

One of the best strategies for assessing intercultural interventions is to ask the client. Because a primary goal of intervention is improved client function and subjective well-being, reports from the client can provide useful feedback. This strategy, known as member checking, allows you to seek specific information regarding choices of intervention, verbal interactions, attempts to demonstrate respect, and factual information about client culture. In fact, even negative interactions can sometimes be turned around through post-intervention reflection with the client or, even better, through frequent checks during the course of intervention.

You might, for example, say to the client, "I said X because I wanted to demonstrate respect for your culture. Did you perceive it in this way?" or "We agreed to intervention Y as a way to help you function in your home environment. Did the intervention help in your situation?" or "What did I say or do that suggested to you that I need to know more about your culture?" This kind of information-seeking may or may not alter the immediate intervention situation but will almost certainly enhance the clinician's ability to be more effective in subsequent interactions.

Meta-Ethnography: Doing Ethnography on Yourself

A final way for you as a health care provider to monitor and assess your behaviors is to view yourself as an ethnographic subject, just as you have learned to view your clients. Thinking of yourself in this way can help keep you from feeling too defensive or being too self-critical. All clinicians, just like all other human beings, including ethnographers, make mistakes. They react too quickly or make inaccurate assumptions. They forget how much their own cultural vantage conditions their responses and behaviors. Even with the best intentions and the desire at all times to provide the best possible service, they may blame the patient or be blind to the ways in which client, system, and practitioner values can collide. All these realities are part of being human. They must be kept in mind but cannot be allowed to paralyze us. They are best thought of as indications of where we need further work on issues of cultural awareness. One way to remind ourselves of that reality is to think of ourselves as equal actors with the client in a cultural drama. We are also potential sources of cultural data.

Whenever you are doing all the other forms of self-evaluation, you can practice viewing your own behaviors with the same stance of careful observation, insightful interpretation, and ongoing inquiry that you are learning to apply to the therapeutic encounter in general. Reflect on your own motives. Consider your own cultural, experiential, professional contexts and think about how they may influence your behavior at a particular point in an interaction or in your patterns of referring to a client even when the client is not present.

If the client seems noncompliant, for example, inspect your own assumptions and interactions to see whether the label is being properly applied. Very few clients are truly trying to undermine their own care. Usually a situation of noncompliance results from a lack of fit between the client's perceptions of what needs to be done, how to do it, or why and the provider's perceptions. That is, it is a failure of effective accommodation. Thinking of yourself as an ethnographic subject can help you evaluate your own perceptions in a more objective way, just as you are trying to learn to evaluate your clients' perceptions without stereotyping or misunderstanding.

Once you adopt an ethnographic mindset, you are likely to be less judgmental and more curious about others. You will also become more objective and insightful about your own behavior. As in doing ethnography with your clients, doing ethnography on yourself is a long, evolving process. You are always learning. One of us had the experience of conducting a lengthy period of field research in a remote area where she lived with people who had ideas about animals and human relationships with animals that were very different from her own. The process of identifying her own assumptions, emotions, and reactions to observations and encounters involving animals around the house only began in the field. It was not fully processed until some 4 years later when she wrote about the experience (Martin, 1990). By that time, she had come to realize how unusual her own behavior must have seemed to others and how badly she had misinterpreted the behavior of others. This delay is natural and will happen to you, too.

One of the best strategies for coping with a process like this one is to maintain a journal in which your dilemmas, discomforts, insights, questions, and self-assessments can be kept, revisited, and used for later reflection. Just as you make ethnographic notes about your interactions with clients for professional purposes, make some about yourself. You will see over time how your reactions to the process and your experiences with the application of the principles you are learning here will transform your understanding of all interactions.

8-15. If you have been keeping a journal for the course or project for which you are reading this book, pause here and reread your journal. Summarize any changes you observe in your attitudes or actions, as recorded in your journal. Are your beliefs the same now as when you began?

Q

ELEMENTS OF CULTURALLY INCLUSIVE THERAPY

Below we summarize the arguments from the preceding chapters and delineate our conclusions and suggestions for practice. Experienced clinicians may find little that is new or different from traditional good practice procedures, and this finding is reassuring. Our goal has not been to redefine health care, only to make the cultural component of health care practices more explicit and thus to prepare a foundation for responsive theory.

The five elements for culturally inclusive health care indicated below are logically ordered statements that prepare one for the practice of culturally inclusive therapy. If you recognize the utility of these statements, believe them, and attempt to put them into practice, you will be better prepared to care for clients whose culture differs substantially from your own. Of course, they also are appropriate in dealing with clients whose cultural background seems similar to your own.

The Conception of Quality of Life

The conception of quality of life—and of its antagonist, an unwanted condition—rests fundamentally with the client. Cultural factors, the client's culture emergent, always affect such conceptions, and the clinician should respect the client's views and work within the cultural frame of the client to the extent possible.

Hahn (1995) has written persuasively about the nature of sickness across cultures. Broadly speaking, the essence of sickness is an unwanted condition in one's person or self—one's mind, body, soul, or connection to the world. What counts as sickness is thus determined by the perception and experience of its bearer, the patient. Sicknesses represent and express the particularities of individual patients within a society. What defines the event for which we seek a cause, however, may be not the patient's body, behaviors, or potentially harmful environmental occurrences—its possible causes—but rather his or her subjective experience and values.

Kleinman et al. (1978) have described what they call the explanatory models that health professionals and clients bring to the clinical encounter. The explanatory model is the way in which persons understand sickness or unwanted conditions. It includes ideas about the causes of those conditions, the circumstances of their onset, how sickness produces its effects, the course of sickness, and possible treatments (Hahn, 1995).

According to Hahn (1995), sicknesses include broken limbs, cancers, and "neurotic" habits that get in one's way. Thus, any of the unwanted conditions that might bring a client to a practitioner would be included in Hahn's definition of sickness.

We agree with Hahn that sickness, along with quality of life and unwanted conditions, is best understood from the perspective of the individual client.

Because of differences in education and other life experiences, the clinician and the client inevitably bring different conceptions of quality of life and of the nature of unwanted conditions to the health care encounter. Ultimately, however, it is the client's conception that must be primary. The client is the one who chooses to comply with instructions or not; to change his or her lifestyle or not; to summon up courage and motivation or not.

The Social and Cultural Environment

The social and cultural environment plays a critical role in therapy; to ignore these factors may jeopardize the client's recovery. You cannot safely make assumptions about the client's environment, especially for clients with a different cultural orientation than yours. Remember that each interaction with a client is an opportunity to learn more about his or her environment. Relationships and cultural beliefs may themselves be healthful or unhealthful, therapeutic or pathogenic. For example, people who are connected socially to others have lower mortality rates, indicating that social connectedness may be a precursor to, rather than a result of, good health (Hahn, 1995). Clinicians have long recognized a parallel reality—those patients with social support networks are better candidates for therapy than those who are socially isolated.

All Therapy Is Intercultural

There is individual variability among all clinicians and all clients; part of this variability is cultural. Clients and clinicians inevitably conceive of the world, communicate, and behave in ways that cannot be assumed to be similar or readily compatible (Hahn, 1995). Measured in terms of patient compliance or satisfaction, the successful health care provider therefore must *prima facie* be an astute ethnographer of his or her clients (Stein, 1982).

Humans are born into societies that inform them how the world is and how to behave in it. People born into one society are likely to have views of the world and of proper behavior very different from the views of people born into another society. In part because they see the world differently, in part because what they see is different, they live in different worlds (Hahn, 1995).

Therapy Is a Social Activity

Health care is a social activity, and the clinician is a facilitator. The clinician–client relationship is the most important aspect of health care (Stein, 1982), and developing this relationship with clients who do not share your cultural orientation requires special considerations. As Saunders (1954) has written with respect to physicians,

> The social relationship is not something apart from medical practice which, like the icing on a cake, can be included or left out at the discretion of the practitioner. It is rather an integral and necessary part of medical practice, without which there is no practice. (p. 243)

The social relationship is no less important, and arguably it is more important, for other health care providers—such as therapists, nurses, social workers, and psychologists—than for physicians.

Come to know your client: establish rapport, understand the client's condition, recognize the client's goals, assess effective modes of therapy, and gain the client's loyalty and confidence. As Hahn (1995) has noted, "Skills in understanding the patient's circumstances and perspective on a condition may be necessary to understand and treat the condition and satisfy the patient" (p. 290).

Try to understand the full context of the client's situation; the focus should be on the client's life, not just the clinical condition. As you interact with your clients, evaluate them, and direct them, you are implicitly conducting an ethnographic inquiry (Stein, 1982).

The objective is to understand the client's explanatory model, as well as the social and cultural factors that may have affected the client's condition and may affect his or her future improvement. Having reached such an understanding, the practitioner will be in a better position to articulate his or her own explanatory model and then discuss the differences and similarities between the two models with the client before negotiating an intervention approach to the client's condition (Hahn, 1995; Katon & Kleinman, 1981).

Use your professional knowledge to help the client move toward his or her expressed goals. The client and the clinician often have different models to explain the client's unwanted condition. It is the clinician's responsibility to translate these differences in ways the client can appreciate.

Respect the client and his or her wishes and concerns. The success of health care depends on the client and clinician working together, and there must be mutual respect before this can occur. The clinician who does not respect cultural norms of interaction may be ineffective in explaining conditions or treatments to clients and may fail to achieve the client's acceptance of recommended interventions (Hahn, 1995). Demonstration of respect for the client may lead to better compliance and thus, in the long run, to better outcomes and greater satisfaction.

It may be necessary to help clients clarify their own values in the process of reaching decisions about care, yet still have the respect not to decide for clients what is in their best interests. As the anthropologist Sol Tax concluded, assume you will never understand them that well (Hinshaw, 1979). Moreover, clinicians should resist the temptation to control encounters with clients. A practitioner has only as much power as the client chooses to delegate. Trust and respect will increase the client's willingness to give the provider additional power. When the clinician and client work together, each surrenders some control so that he or she may reach mutual accommodation.

A Clinician's Education Is Lifelong

Each client is unique—you must begin anew with each one. Culture evolves continuously; thus, so will clients' and clinicians' conceptions of quality of life, unwanted conditions, and the value of particular interventions. The role of the clinician is to understand the client's condition and circumstances, to develop knowledge and techniques, to communicate this knowledge and expertise to clients, and to apply this knowledge for the assistance of clients in achieving their own goals (Hahn, 1995). Thus, there is always more to learn, more to do.

Health care is full of ambiguity, and culture is only one ambiguous element with which clinicians must deal. Uncertainty about evaluations or interventions, whether one has done enough to ensure the establishment of a collaborative plan, whether one should do more to assist the client in nontherapeutic ways (e.g., with social services) to improve healthfulness—these are only some of the many ambiguities clinicians continuously face. Cultural unknowns are just one more.

Although formal education in the form of professional coursework and continuing education can help and may be essential to address the issue, the education that comes from experience and from continuously rejecting stereotypes and traditional assumptions is also important. Doing ethnographies of your clients can be an especially enlightening educational undertaking.

Include the lessons from this text in your professional practice and that practice will be more culturally inclusive, with potentially better outcomes for all your clients. In addition, you will enjoy working with a wider range of clients, and you will continue to learn about different cultures and to appreciate cultural differences. You may even find that you have a greater overall sense of professional pride because you are providing better services to all types of clients. We wish you great success in this important enterprise.

✎ NOTES ✐

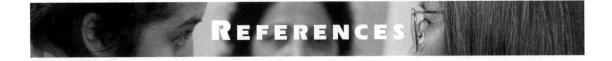

REFERENCES

Agar, M. H. (1996). *The professional stranger: An informal introduction to ethnography*. San Diego, CA: Academic Press.

Allman, A. (1990). *Subjective well-being of people with disabilities: Measurement issues*. Unpublished master's thesis, University of Illinois, Chicago.

Allotey, T., Nikles, J., & Manderson, L. (1998). *Cultural division guidelines to practice* [On-line]. Available: http://www.health.qld.gov.au/

Alvord, L. A., & Van Pelt, E. C. (1999). *The scalpel and the silver bear: The first Navajo woman surgeon combines Western medicine and traditional healing*. New York: Bantam.

American Medical Association. (1999). *Cultural competence compendium*. Chicago: Author.

American Medical Student Association. (1999). *Cultural competency in medicine* [On-line]. Available: http://www.amsa.org/programs/gpit/cultural.htm

American Occupational Therapy Association. (1999). *Standards for accreditation of an occupational therapy educational program*. Rockville, MD: Author.

American Psychiatric Association. (1994). *Diagnostic and statistical manual of mental disorders* (4th ed.) Washington, DC: Author.

American Psychological Association. (1993). APA guidelines for providers of psychological services to ethnic, linguistic, and culturally diverse populations. *American Psychologist, 48*, 45-48.

American Psychological Association. (2000). *Annual conference program.* [On-line]. Available: http://www.apa.org/conf.html

American Speech and Hearing Association. (1999). *Annual conference program.* [On-line]. Available: http://www.asha.org

Angier, N. (2000, August 22). Do races differ? Not really, DNA shows. *New York Times*. Retrieved from http://www.nytimes.com

Arnett, F. C., Edworthy, S. M., Bloch, D. A., McShane, D. J., Fries, J. F., Cooper, N. S., Healey, L. A., Kaplan, S. R., Liang, M. H. & Luthra, H. S. (1988). The American Rheumatism Association 1987 revised criteria for the classification of rheumatoid arthritis. *Arthritis and Rheumatology, 31*, 315-324.

Arnett, J. J. (1999). Adolescent storm and stress, reconsidered. *American Psychologist, 54*, 317-326.

Bandlamudi, L. (1994). Dialogics of understanding self/culture. *Ethos, 22*, 460-493.

Banks, C. G. (1992). "Culture" in culture-bound syndromes: The case of anorexia nervosa. *Social Science and Medicine, 34*, 867-884.

Bates, M. S., & Edwards, W. T. (1992). Ethnic variations in chronic pain experience. *Ethnicity and Disease, 2*, 63-83.

Bechtel, G. A., Davidhizar, R., & Bunting, S. (2000). Triangulation research among culturally diverse populations. *Journal of Allied Health, 29*, 61-63.

Belay, G. (1996). The reconstruction and negotiation of cultural identities in the age of globalization. In H. B. Mokros (Ed.), *Interaction and identity: Information and behavior*. New Brunswick, NJ: Transaction.

Bell, R. (1995). Prominence of women in Navajo healing beliefs and values. *Nursing Health Care, 15*, 232-242.

Belliotti, R. A. (1993). *Good sex: A perspective on sexual ethics*. Lawrence, KS: University of Kansas Press.

Bernstein, C. N. (1999). Placebos in medicine. *Seminars in Gastrointestinal Disease, 10*, 3-7.

Blakeslee, S. (1998, October 13). Placebos prove so powerful even experts are surprised. *New York Times*. Retrieved from http://www.nytimes.com

Blum, D. (1997). *Sex on the brain: The biological differences between men and women*. New York: Penguin Press.

Bohannon, P., & Van der Eist, D. (1998). *Asking and listening: Ethnography, a personal adaptation*. Prospect Heights, IL: Waveland Press.

Briggs, C. L. (1986). *Learning how to ask*. Cambridge, MA: Cambridge University Press.

Brody, J. E. (2000, April 25). Personal health: Memories of things that never were. *New York Times*. Retrieved from http://www.nytimes.com

Brown, P. J. (1998). *Understanding and applying medical anthropology*. Mountain View, CA: Mayfield.

Bruner, J. (1987). Life as narrative. *Social Research, 54*, 11-32.

Brunstein, J. D. (1993). Personal goals and subjective well-being. *Journal of Personality and Social Psychology, 65*, 1061-1070.

Burns, A. F. (1993). *Maya in exile: Guatemalans in Florida*. Philadelphia: Temple University Press.

Callahan, J. (1989). *Don't worry, he won't get far on foot: The autobiography of a dangerous man*. New York: Morrow.

Camphina-Bacote, J. (1999). A model and instrument for addressing cultural competence in health care. *Journal of Nursing Education, 38*, 203-206.

Carrithers, M. (1992). *Why humans have cultures: Explaining anthropology and social diversity*. Oxford, England: Oxford University Press.

Cerroni-Long, E. L. (2000). Through the multiculturalism window. *Anthropology News, 41*(1), 9-10.

Chapple, E. D. (1970). *Culture and biological man*. New York: Holt.

Chapple, E. D., & Coon, C. S. (1942). *Principles of anthropology*. New York: Holt.

Clifton, J. (1976). Mazeway. In D. E. Hunter & P. Whitten (Eds.), *Encyclopedia of anthropology* (pp. 262-263). New York: Harper & Row.

Colapinto, J. (2000). *As nature made him: The boy who was raised as a girl*. New York: Harpercollins.

Collins, W. A., Maccoby, E. E., Steinberg, L., Hetherington, E. M., & Bornstein, M. H. (2000). Contemporary research on parenting: The case for nature and nurture. *American Psychologist, 55*, 218-232.

Commission on Accreditation of Physical Therapy Education. (1998). *Evaluative criteria for accreditation of educational programs for the preparation of physical therapists*. Washington, DC: Author.

Cousins, N. (1979). *Anatomy of an illness as perceived by the patient*. New York: Norton.

Crabtree, B. F., & Miller, W. L. (1999). *Doing qualitative research*. Thousand Oaks, CA: Sage.

Craik, C., & Alderman, J. J. (1998). What attracts mature students to occupational therapy? *British Journal of Occupational Therapy, 61*, 473-477.

Crigger, B. J. (Ed.). (1998). *Cases in bioethics: Selections from the Hastings Center Report.* Boston: Bedford/St. Martin's.

Csikszentmihalyi, M. (1975). *Beyond boredom and anxiety.* San Francisco: Jossey–Bass.

Cuellar, I., & Arnold, B. R. (1988). Cultural considerations and rehabilitation of disabled Mexican Americans. *Journal of Rehabilitation, 54,* 35-41.

D'Aquili, E. G., Laughlin, C. D., & McManus, J. (1979). *The spectrum of ritual.* New York: Columbia University Press.

Dana, R. H. (1998). *Understanding cultural identity in intervention and assessment.* Thousand Oaks, CA: Sage.

Davis, D. (1994). It ain't necessarily so: Clinicians, bioethics, and religious studies. *Journal of Clinical Ethics, 5,* 315-319.

Davis, D. S. (2000). Groups, communities, and contested identities in genetic research. *Hastings Center Report, 30,* 38-45.

Davis, R. (1989). *My journey into Alzheimer's disease.* Wheaton, IL: Tyndale House.

DeVoe, D., Kennedy, C., & Pena, M. (1998). Health promotion students: Background profiles and occupational decision factors. *College Student Journal, 32,* 197-202.

Diener, E., Suh, E., & Oishi, S. (1997). Recent findings on subjective well-being. *Indian Journal of Clinical Psychology, 24,* 25-41.

DiversityRx. (1997a). *Multicultural best practices* [On-line]. Available: http://www.DiversityRx.org/BEST/index.html

DiversityRx. (1997b). *Why language and culture are important* [On-line]. Available: http://www.DiversityRx.org/HTML/ESLANG.htm

Draper, P., & Harpending, H. (1994). Cultural considerations in the experience of aging: Two African cultures. In B. R. Bonder & M. B. Wagner (Eds.), *Functional performance in older adults* (pp. 15-27). Philadelphia: F.A. Davis.

Durante, A. (1997). *Linguistic anthropology.* Cambridge: Cambridge University Press.

Ellin, A. (2000, June 6). High-tech philanthropy in a low-tech Guatemalan village. *New York Times.* Retrieved from http://www.nytimes.com

Ellis, A., & Harper, R. A. (1961). *A guide to rational living.* (p. 88). Hollywood, CA: Wilshire Book Co.

Ellis, B. B., & Kimmel, H. D. (1992). Identification of unique cultural response patterns by means of item response theory. *Journal of Applied Psychology, 77,* 177-184.

Emerson, R. M. (1983). *Contemporary field research: A collection of readings.* Boston: Little, Brown.

England, J. (1986). Cross-cultural heath care. *Canada's Mental Health, 34*(4), 13-15.

Fadiman, A. (1997). *The spirit catches you and you fall down.* New York: Noonday Press.

Fazio, S., Seman, D., & Stansell, J. (1999). *Rethinking Alzheimer's care.* Baltimore: Health Professions Press.

Feldman, K. W. (1995). Pseudoabusive burns in a Somali child. *Child Abuse and Neglect, 19,* 657-658.

Fortier, J. P. (1999). *Multicultural health best practices overview* [On-line]. Available: http://www.DiversityRx.org/BEST/index.html.

Foster, G. M., & Anderson, B. G. (1978). *Medical anthropology.* New York: Wiley.

Freeman, J., & Loewe, R. (2000). Barriers to communication about diabetes mellitus. Patients' and physicians' different view of the disease. *Journal of Family Practice, 49,* 507-512.

French, H. W. (2000, May 3). Japan unsettles returnees who yearn to leave again. *New York Times.* Retrieved from http://www.nytimes.com

Freud, S. (1900/1965). Obsessive acts and religious practices. In W. A. Lessa & E. Z. Vogt (Eds.), *Reader in comparative religion: An anthropological approach* (2nd ed., pp. 185-190). New York: Harper & Row.

Funder, D. C. (1997). *The personality puzzle.* New York: Norton.

Galanti, G. (1997). *Caring for patients from different cultures: Case studies from American hospitals* (2nd ed.). Philadelphia: University of Pennsylvania Press.

Geertz, C. (1984). From the native's point of view: On the nature of anthropological understanding. In R. A. Shweder & R. LeVine (Eds.), *Culture theory: Essays on mind, self, and emotion.* Cambridge, MA: Cambridge University Press.

Giger, J. N., & Davidhizar, R. E. (1991). *Transcultural nursing: Assessment and intervention.* St. Louis: Mosby.

Gluckman, M., & Gluckman, M. (1977). On drama and games and athletic contests. In S. P. Moore & B. Myerhoff (Eds.), *Secular ritual* (pp. 227-243). Assen, the Netherlands: von Gorcum.

Goode, E. (2000, August 8). How culture molds habits of thought. *New York Times.*

Retrieved from http://www.nytimes.com

Goode, M. (2000, March 14). Human nature: Born or made? *New York Times.* Retrieved from http://www.nytimes.com

Goody, J., & Watt, I. (1963). The consequences of literacy. *Comparative Studies in Society and History, 5,* 3.

Grbich, C. (1998). *Qualitative research in health: An introduction.* Thousand Oaks, CA: Sage.

Hahn, R. A. (1995). *Sickness and healing: An anthropological perspective.* New Haven, CT: Yale University Press.

Hammer, M. R. (1998). A measure of intercultural sensitivity: The Intercultural Development Inventory. In S. Fowler & M. Fowler (Eds.), *The intercultural sourcebook* (Vol. 2). Yarmouth, ME: Intercultural Press.

Harris, C. H. (2000, March 13). Educating toward multiculturalism. *OT Practice, 5,* 7-8.

Harris, S. L. (2000). Pervasive developmental disorders: The spectrum of autism. In M. Hersen & R. T. Ammerman (Eds.), *Advanced abnormal child psychology* (2nd ed., pp. 357-370). Mahwah, NJ: Erlbaum.

Hashimoto, A. (1996). *The gift of generations: Japanese and American perspectives on aging and the social contract.* Cambridge, MA: Cambridge University Press.

Health Care Financing Administration. (1999). *Minimum Data Set (MDS)—Version 2.0.* Washington, DC: Author.

Hennessy, C. H., & John, R. (1995). The interpretation of burden among Pueblo Indian caregivers. *Journal of Aging Studies, 9,* 215-229.

Hill, J. H., & MacLaurey, R. E. (1995). The terror of Montezuma: Aztec history, vantage theory, and the category of 'person.' In J. R. Taylor & R. MacLaurey (Eds.), *Language and the cognitive construal of the world. Trends in linguistics, Studies and monographs 82* (pp. 277-329). Berlin, Germany: Mouton de Gruyter.

Hill, R. F., & Fortenberry, J. D. (1992). Adolescence as a culture-bound syndrome. *Social Science and Medicine, 35*, 73-80.

Hinshaw, R. (Ed.). (1979). *Currents in anthropology: Essays in honor of Sol Tax*. The Hague, the Netherlands: Mouton.

Hoff, T. J. (1998). Same profession, different people: Stratification, structure, and physicians? Employment choices. *Sociological Forum, 13*, 133-156.

Hojat, M. J., Brigham, T. P., Gottheil, E., Xu, G., Glaser, K., & Veloski, J. J. (1998). Medical students? Personal values and their career choices a quarter-century later. *Psychological Reports, 83*, 243-248.

Hong, Y., Morris, M. W., Chiu, C., & Benet-Martinez, V. (2000). Multicultural minds: A dynamic constructivist approach to culture and cognition. *American Psychologist, 55*, 709-720.

Horgan, J. (1996). *The undiscovered mind. How the human brain defies replication, medication, and explanation*. New York: The Free Press.

Hrobjartsson, A., & Gotzsche, P. C. (2001). Is the placebo powerless? An analysis of clinical trials comparing placebos with no treatment. *The New England Journal of Medicine, 344*, 1594-1602.

Hughes, C. C., & Okpaku, S. O. (1998). Culture's role in clinical and psychiatric assessment. In S. O. Okpaku (Ed.), *Clinical methods in transcultural psychiatry* (pp. 213-232). Washington, DC: American Psychiatric Association Press.

James, S. A. (2000). *Racial and ethnic differences in infant mortality: A sociocultural analysis*. Presented at the National Institutes of Health Conference, Toward Higher Levels of Analysis: Progress and Promise in Research on Social and Cultural Aspects of Health, Bethesda, MD.

Janesick, V. J. (1998). *"Stretching" exercises for qualitative researchers*. Thousand Oaks, CA: Sage.

Jibaja, M. L., Sebastian, R., Kingery, P., & Holcomb, J. D. (2000). The multicultural sensitivity of physician assistant students. *Journal of Allied Health, 29*, 79-85.

Johnson, T. M., Hardt, E., & Kleinman, A. (1995). Cultural factors in the medical interview. In M. Lipkin, S. M. Putnam, & A. Lazare (Eds.), *The medical interview: Clinical care, education, and research* (pp. 153-162). New York: Springer–Verlag.

Katon, W., & Kleinman, A. (1981). Doctor–patient negotiations and other social science strategies in patient care. In L. Eisenberg & A. Kleinman (Eds.), *The relevance of social science for medicine*. Boston: D. Reidel.

Kim, Y. Y. (1996). Identity development: From cultural to intercultural. In H. B. Mokros (Ed.), *Interaction and identity* (pp. 347-369). New Brunswick, NJ: Transaction Publications.

Kleinman, A. (1980). *Patients and healers in the context of culture: An exploration of the borderland between anthropology, medicine, and psychiatry*. Berkeley, CA: University of California Press.

Kleinman, A. M., Eisenberg, L., & Good, B. (1978). Culture, illness, and care. *Annals of Internal Medicine, 88*, 251-258.

Kluckhohn, F. R., & Strodtbeck, F. L. (1961). *Variations in value orientations*. Evanston, IL: Row, Peterson.

Koyano, W. (1989). Japanese attitudes toward the elderly: A review of research findings. *Journal of Cross-Cultural Gerontology, 4*, 335-345.

Krefting, L. (1991). Rigor in qualitative research: The assessment of trustworthiness. *American Journal of Occupational Therapy, 45*, 214-222.

Kreps, G. L., & Kunimoto, E. N. (1994). *Effective communication in multicultural health care settings*. Thousand Oaks, CA: Sage.

Kubler-Ross, E. (1968). *On death and dying*. New York: McMillan.

Kushner, H. S. (1992). *When bad things happen to good people*. New York: Avon Books.

Laughlin, C. D. Jr., McManus, J., & d'Aquili, E. G. (1992). *Brain, symbol and experience: Toward a neurophenomenology of human consciousness*. New York: Columbia University Press.

Law, M. (1998). *Client-centered occupational therapy*. Thorofare, NJ: SLACK Incorporated.

Le Postallec, M. (1999, November 22). Being competent with culture. *ADVANCE for Physical Therapists & PT Assistants*, 6-13.

Lewicki, E. L., Smith, S. L., Cash, S. H., Madigan, M. S., & Simons, D. F. (1999). Factors influencing practice area preference in occupational therapy. *Occupational Therapy in Mental Health, 12*, 1-19.

Lex, B. W. (1979). The neurobiology of ritual trance. In E. G. d'Aquili, C. D. Laughlin, Jr., & Y. J. McManus (Eds.), *The spectrum of ritual* (pp. 117-182). New York: Columbia University Press.

Loveland, C. A. (1999). The concept of culture. In R. L. Leavitt (Ed.), *Cross-cultural rehabilitation: An international perspective* (pp. 15-24). London: Saunders.

Low, B. S. (1999). *Why sex matters. A Darwinian look at human behavior*. Princeton, NJ: Princeton University Press.

Luborsky, M. (1994). The cultural adversity of physical disability: Erosion of full adult personhood. *Journal of Aging Studies, 8*, 239-253.

Lynn, S. J., & McConkey, K. M. (Eds.). (1998). *Truth in memory*. New York: Guilford Press.

Ma, G. X. (2000). Barriers to the use of health services by Chinese Americans. *Journal of Allied Health, 29*, 64-70.

MacLaurey, R. (1997). *Color and cognition in Mesoamerica: Constructing categories as vantages*. Austin: University of Texas Press.

Malcomson, S. L. (2000). *One drop of blood: The American misadventure of race*. New York: Farrar Straus & Giroux.

Marshall, P. A. (1992). Anthropology and bioethics. *Medical Anthropology Quarterly, 6*, 49-73.

Marshall, P. A., & Koenig, B. A. (1996). Bioethics in anthropology: Perspectives on culture, medicine, and morality. In C. F. Sargent & T. M. Johnson (Eds.), *Medical anthropology: Contemporary theory and method* (Rev. ed., pp. 349-373). Westport, CT: Praeger.

Martin, L. (1990). Beasts of the field. *Anthropology and Humanism Quarterly, 15*(2/3), 38-49.

Masden, W. (1955). Hot and cold in the universe of San Francisco Tecospa, Valley of Mexico. *Journal of American Folklore, 68*, 123-139.

Masi, R., & Disman, M. (1994). Health care and seniors: Ethnic, racial, and cultural dimensions. *Canadian Family Physician, 40*, 498-504.

Massimini, F., & Fave, A. D. (2000). Individual development in a bio-cultural perspective. *American Psychologist, 55*(1), 24-33.

Mattingly, C. (1998). *Healing dramas and clinical plots: The narrative structure of experience*. Cambridge, MA: Cambridge University Press.

Mattson, S., & Lew, L. (1991). Culturally sensitive prenatal care for Southeast Asians. *Journal of Obstetrical, Gynecological, and Neonatal Nursing, 12,* 48-54.

McClure, F. H., & Teyber, E. (1996). The multicultural–relational approach. In F. H. McClure & E. Teyber (Eds.), *Child and adolescent therapy: A multicultural–relational approach* (pp. 1-32). Ft. Worth, TX: Harcourt Brace.

McCullough, J. M. (1973). Human ecology, heat adaptation, and belief systems: The hot–cold syndrome of Yucatan. *Journal of Anthropological Research, 29*(1), 32-36.

McElroy, A., & Townsend, P. A. (Eds.). *Medical anthropology in ecological perspective* (3rd ed.). Boulder, CO: Westview.

Miller, J. G. (1997). Agency and context in cultural psychology: Implications for moral theory. In H. D. Saltzstein (Ed.), *Culture as a context for moral development: New perspectives on the particular and the universal* (pp. 69-85). San Francisco: Jossey–Bass.

Miller, J., & Bersoff, D. M. (1992). Culture and moral judgment: How are conflicts between justice and interpersonal responsibility resolved? *Journal of Personality and Social Psychology, 62,* 541-554.

Miner, H. (1956). Body ritual among the Nacirema. *American Anthropologist, 58,* 503-507.

Miracle, A. W. (1997). A shaman to organizations. In C. R. Ember, M. Ember, & P. N. Peregrine (Eds.), *Research frontiers in anthropology* (Vol. 1, pp. 133-150). Englewood Cliffs, NJ: Prentice Hall.

Miracle, A. W., & Southard, D. (1993). The athlete and ritual timing: An experimental study. *Journal of Ritual Studies, 7*(1), 125-138.

Miracle, C. S. (1981). Intelligence testing and the Aymara. In M. J. Hardman (ed.). *The Aymara language in its social and cultural context.* (pp. 240-247). Gainesville: University Presses of Florida.

Murphy, R. (1981). Review of the Way of the shaman: A guide to power and healing by Michael Harner. *American Anthropologist, 83,* 714-717.

Murphy, R. F. (1987). *The body silent.* New York: Holt.

National Institute on Disability and Rehabilitation Research, Office of Special Education and Rehabilitative Services. (1993). Culturally sensitive rehabilitation. Bringing research into effective focus. *Rehab Brief, 15*(8).

Nayak, S., Shiflett, S. C., Eshun, S., & Levine, F. M. (2000). Culture and gender effects in pain beliefs and the prediction of pain tolerance. *Cross-Cultural Research, 34,* 135-151.

Neff, N. (1997). *Folk medicine in Hispanics in the southwestern United States* [On-line]. Available: http://www.spb.bcm.tmc.edu/HispanicHealth/Courses/mod7/mod7.html

Neugarten, B. L., Havighurst, R. J., & Tobin, S. S. (1961). The measurement of life satisfaction. *Journal of Gerontology, 16,* 134-143.

New waves: Hospitals struggle to meet the challenge of multiculturalism now—and in the next generation. (1993). *Hospitals, 67,* 22-31.

Nichter, M. (2000). *Sociocultural factors influencing tobacco use, nicotine dependency and smoking cessation: How global and North American studies can inform each other.* Presented at the National Institutes of Health Conference Toward Higher Levels of Analysis: Progress and Promise in Research on Social and Cultural Dimensions of Health, Bethesda, MD.

Nisbett, R. E., Peng, K., Choi, I., & Norenzayan, A. (2001). Culture and systems of thought: Holistic vs. analytic cognition. *Psychological Review, 108,* 291-310.

Nobel, J., & Lacasa, J. (1991). *The Hispanic way: Aspects of behavior, attitudes, and customs in the Spanish-speaking world.* Lincolnwood, IL: Passport Books.

Nolan, K. (1998). Live sperm, dead bodies. In B. J. Crigger (Ed.), *Cases in bioethics: Selections from the Hastings Center Report* (p. 69). Boston: Bedford/St. Martin's.

Nucci, L. (1997). Culture, universals, and the personal. In H. D. Saltzstein (Ed.), *Culture as a context for moral development: New perspectives on the particular and the universal* (pp. 5-22). San Francisco: Jossey–Bass.

Office of Minority Health. (2000). *Assuring cultural competence in health care: Recommendations for national standards and an outcomes-focused research agenda.* Washington, DC: U.S. Public Health Service.

Okun, M. S., Stock, W. A., Haring, M. J., & Witter, R. A. (1984). The social activity/subjective well-being relation: A quantitative synthesis. *Research on Aging, 6,* 45-65.

Orlansky, M. D., & Heward, W. L. (1981). *Voices: Interviews with handicapped people.* Columbus, OH: Charles E. Merrill.

Osterweis, M., McLaughlin, C. J., Manasse, H. R., & Hopper, C. L. (Eds.). (1996). *The U.S. health workforce: Power, politics, and policy.* Washington, DC: Association of Academic Health Centers.

Pavot, W., & Diener, E. (1993). The affective and cognitive context of self-reported measures of subjective well-being. *Social Indicators Research, 24,* 35-56.

Peng, K., & Nisbett, R. E. (1999). Culture, dialectics, and reasoning about contradiction. *American Psychologist, 54,* 741-754.

Peoples, J., & Bailey, G. (1997). *Humanity: An introduction to cultural anthropology* (4th ed.). Belmont, CA: West Wadsworth.

Physician's Weekly. (2000). *Are cultural competence activities worthwhile?* [On-line]. Available: http://www.physweekly.com/pc.html

Pimental, F. L., Ferreira, J. S., Real, M. V., Mesquita, N. F., & Maia-Goncalves, J. P. (1999, September 9). Quantity and quality of information desired by Portuguese cancer patients. *Support Care Cancer, 7,* 407-412.

Pittler, E. R. (1999). Experts' opinions on complementary/alternative therapies for low back pain. *Journal of Manipulative Physical Therapy, 22,* 87-90.

Power, M., Bullinger, M., Harper, A., & The World Health Organization Quality of Life Group. (1999). The World Health Organization WHOQOL-100: Tests of the universality of quality of life in 15 different cultural groups worldwide. *Health Psychology, 18*(5), 495-505.

Pruegger, V. J., & Rogers, T. B. (1994). Cross-cultural sensitivity training: Methods and assessment. *International Journal of Intercultural Relations, 18,* 369-387.

Purnell, L. D., & Paulanka, B. J. (1998). Transcultural diversity and health care. In L. D. Purnell & B. J. Paulanka (Eds.), *Transcultural health care: A culturally competent approach* (pp. 1-6). Philadelphia: F.A. Davis.

Queensland Government. (1998, November). *Guidelines to practice* [On-line]. Available: http://www.health.qld.gov.au

Radomski, M. V. (1995). Nationally speaking, there is more to life than putting on your pants. *American Journal of Occupational Therapy, 49*(6), 487-490.

Rakos, R. (1999, May). Control and countercontrol in the therapeutic relationship: Ethical and legal issues for behavioral clinicians. Presented at the annual convention of the Association for Behavior Analysts, Chicago, IL.

Ramos, J. (2000). *What it really takes to improve cultural competency. The Center for Multicultural and Multilingual Mental Health Services.* [Online] Available: http://www.mcmlmhs.org/cultures/issueessays/really.htm

Reese, D. J., Ahern, R. E., Nair, S., O'Faire, J. D., & Warren, C. (1999). Hospice access and use by African-Americans: Addressing cultural and institutional barriers through participatory action research. *Social Work, 44,* 549-559.

Rogler, L. H. (1999). Methodological sources of cultural insensitivity in mental health research. *American Psychologist, 54,* 424-433.

Rossman, G. B., & Rallis, S. F. (1998). *Learning in the field: An introduction to qualitative research.* Thousand Oaks, CA: Sage.

Rowles, G. D. (1991). Beyond performance: Being in place as a component of occupational therapy. *American Journal of Occupational Therapy, 45,* 265-271.

Rubin, H. J., & Rubin, I. S. (1995). *Qualitative interviewing: The art of hearing data.* Thousand Oaks, CA: Sage.

Sacks, O. (1989). *Seeing voices: A journey into the world of the deaf.* Berkeley, CA: University of California Press.

Saunders, L. (1954). *Cultural difference and medical care: The care of Spanish-speaking people of the Southwest.* New York: Russell Sage.

Scheer, J., & Luborsky, M. (1991). The cultural context of polio biographies. *Orthopedics, 14,* 1173-1181.

Seelman, K. D. (1999). *The new paradigm of disability envisions disabled people as citizens living independently in their communities* [On-line]. Available: http://www.accessiblesociety.org/bkgdcinidrlrp.htm

Sharon, D. (1978). *Wizard of the four winds: A shaman's story.* New York: The Free Press.

Sherzer, J. A. (1987). Discourse-centered approach to language and culture. *American Anthropologist, 89,* 295-309.

Silver, R. L. (1980). *Coping with an undesirable life event: A study of early reactions to physical disability.* Unpublished doctoral dissertation, Northwestern University, Evanston, IL.

Sleek, S. (1998, December). Psychology's cultural competence, once 'simplistic,' now broadening. *APA Monitor, 29*(12), 1, 27.

Sodowsky, G. R., Taffe, R. C., Gutkin, T. B., & Wise, S. L. (1994). Development of the Multicultural Counseling Inventory: A self-report measure of multicultural competencies. *Journal of Counseling Psychology, 4,* 137-148.

Sokolovsky, J. (1997). Aging, family and community development in a Mexican peasant village. In J. Sokolovsky (Ed.), *The cultural context of aging* (pp. 191-217). Westport, CT: Bergin & Garvey.

Spencer, J., Krefting, L., & Mattingly, C. (1993). Incorporation of ethnographic methods in occupational therapy assessment. *American Journal of Occupational Therapy, 47,* 303-309.

Spiegel, D., Bloom, J. R., & Yalom, I. (1981). Group support for patients with metastatic cancer: A randomized prospective outcome study. *Archives of General Psychiatry, 38,* 527-533.

Spokane, A. R. (1992). Personal constructs and careers: A reaction. *Journal of Career Development, 18,* 229-236.

Stein, H. F. (1982). The ethnographic mode of teaching clinical behavior science. In N. J. Chrisman & T. W. Maretzki (Eds.), *Clinically applied anthropology* (pp. 61-86). Boston: D. Reidel.

Stolberg, S. G. (1999, April 25). Sham surgery returns as a research tool. *New York Times.*

Retrieved from http://www.nytimes.com

Sue, S. (2000). *The provision of effective mental health treatment by service providers.* Presented at the National Institutes of Health Conference, Toward Higher Levels of Analysis: Progress and Promise in Research on Social and Cultural Dimensions of Health, Bethesda, MD.

Suh, E., Diener, E., Oishi, S., & Triandis, H. C. (1997). The shifting basis of life satisfaction judgments across cultures: Emotions versus norms. *Journal of Personality and Social Psychology, 74,* 482-493.

Sullivan, L. M., Dukes, K. A., Harris, L., Dittus, R. S., Greenfield, S., & Kaplan, S. H. (1995). A comparison of various methods of collecting self-reported health outcomes data among low-income and minority patients. *Medical Care, 33,* AS183-AS194.

Thomas, S., & Quinn, S. C. (1991). The Tuskegee Syphilis Study, 1932–1972: Implications for HIV education and AIDS risk programs in the black community. *American Journal of Public Health, 81,* 1498-1505.

Tokar, D. M., Fischer, A. R., & Subich, L. M. (1998). Personality and vocational behavior: A selective review of the literature, 1993–1997. *Journal of Vocational Behavior, 53,* 115-153.

A turning-point for AIDS? (2000, July 15). *The Economist, 358,* 77-79.

Urban, G. A. (1991). *Discourse-centered approach to culture: Native South American myths and rituals.* Austin, TX: University of Texas Press.

van Gennep, A. L. (1909/1960). *The rites of passage.* Chicago: University of Chicago Press.

Vygotsky, L. S. (1978). *Mind in society: The development of higher psychological processes.* Cambridge, MA: Harvard University Press.

Wade, N. (2000, May 2). The human family tree: 10 Adams and 18 Eves. *New York Times.*

Retrieved from http://www.nytimes.com

Wainryb, C. (1997). The mismeasure of diversity: Reflections on the study of cross-cultural differences. In H. D. Saltzstein (Ed.), *Culture as a context for moral development. New perspectives on the particular and the universal* (pp. 51-65). San Francisco: Jossey–Bass.

Wallace, A. F. C. (1966). *Religion: An anthropological view.* New York: McGraw-Hill.

Wallace, A. F. C. (1970). *Culture and personality* (2nd ed.). New York: McGraw-Hill.

Ware, J. E., Snow, K. K., Kosinski, M., & Gandek, B. (1993). *36-SF manual and interpretation guide.* Lincoln, RI: Quality Metric.

Wexler, N. E. (1981). Learning to be a leper: A case study in the social construction of illness. In E. G. Mishler (Ed.), *Health, illness and patient care* (pp. 147-157). Cambridge, MA: Cambridge University.

Wiese, H. J. C. (1976). Maternal nutrition and traditional food behavior in Haiti. *Human Organization, 35*(2), 193-200.

Williams, R. M. Jr. (1979). Change and stability in values and value systems: A sociological perspective. In M. Rokeach (Ed.), *Understanding human values: Individual and societal* (pp. 15-46). New York: The Free Press.

Wohl, J. (1989). Integration of cultural awareness into psychotherapy. *American Journal of Psychotherapy, 43*, 343-355.

World Health Organization. (2000). *International Classification of Impairment, Disability, and Handicap* (2nd ed.). Geneva: Author.

Wright, L. (1997). *Twins and what they tell us about who we are.* New York: Wiley.

Yoon, C., Hasher, L., Feinberg, F., Rahhal, T. A., & Winocur, G. (2000). Cross-cultural differences in memory: The role of culture-based stereotypes about aging. *Psychology of Aging, 15*, 694-704.

Zamudio, A. (2000). Finding solutions through the eyes of our patients. *Family Medicine, 32*, 15-16.

GLOSSARY

academic medical centers: large complexes of buildings located in city centers, drawing patients from all over their geographic region (and sometimes beyond), focused on teaching and research in addition to health care.

acculturation: contact between previously autonomous cultural traditions resulting in the adoption of cultural characteristics of each culture by the other.

achieved status: a position in society that is acquired through special effort or competition.

activities of daily living: activities basic to self-maintenance, such as cooking, eating, and self-care.

adaptation: change that occurs as a response to particular environmental circumstances.

alternative explanation: a different way of describing a particular event or experience.

alternative interpretation: a different way of explaining the meaning of a particular event or experience.

ascribed status: a position in society that one acquires by being born into it.

assumptions: beliefs or expectations that predispose one to expect particular events or outcomes, or to interpret events in a particular way.

attitude-centered: an approach to teaching cultural competence focused on valuing of all cultures.

being in becoming orientation: a value orientation found in some cultures that emphasizes activities that have the goal of developing the self.

being orientation: a value orientation found in some cultures in which the preference is for the kind of activity that is a spontaneous expression of the individual human's essence.

bicultural: reflecting characteristics of two primary cultures.

biomedical model: a view of illness that holds that disease always has a definable (usually organic) cause and that medical treatment is the preferred intervention.

bloodless surgery: a surgical approach characterized by various procedures used to minimize blood loss, thereby reducing the need for transfusion.

calendrical rituals: rituals based on annual events such as changes of season, commemoration of specific events, etc.

capacity for surprise: the ability to notice and accept that one's own interpretation is not the only one available.

case conceptualization: a model or theory about a particular health situation based on the individual's assumptions, knowledge, and information gathered about the situation.

cochlear implants: tiny transmitters implanted near the cochlea of a person with a hearing impairment to stimulate transmission of sound from the environment to the brain.

collaterality: social relationship structure defined by laterality.

collectivist: focused on group goals.

communitarian: system in which the good of the group is dominant over the good of individuals.

community hospitals: small health care facilities, usually with inpatient and other kinds of care, located within the community they serve and focused on direct care for relatively uncomplicated conditions.

complex society: a society that includes a large number of cultures.

cross-cultural: interaction between or among individuals of different cultural identities.

cultural broker: a person who serves go-between functions at the edges of cultural groups in contact.

cultural competence: the ability to interact and intervene effectively with individuals from a wide array of cultures.

cultural exclusivity: the existence of a single culture in the absence of all others.

cultural interpreter: a person who is a member of the same group as a client but who is somewhat familiar with American health care procedures, systems, and values.

cultural sensitivity: having respect for and sensitivity to other cultures.

cultural universals: rules, concepts, and strategies for meeting needs that are found in every human group.

culturally inclusive: allowing for multiple cultural perspectives.

culture: "learned patterns of thought and behavior shared by a social group" (Brown, 1998, p. 10).

culture-bound syndromes: "diseases" that seem to be specific to a single culture or a group of related cultures.

culture emergent: a perspective on culture that emphasizes the dynamic, nuanced, and contextual nature of culture.

culture-specific expertise: knowledge of the generally accepted values, beliefs, and behaviors of particular cultural groups (Sue, 2000).

depersonalization: a cognitive process by which the self or others are conceptualized as objects rather than people.

descriptive approach: a method for representing a culture through the systematic identification of the particular traits and material goods of the group.

doing orientation: a value orientation found in some cultures that supports activity as the central focus of existence, with accomplishments measurable by external standards.

dynamic sizing skills: ability to compare widely held views about a culture with the specifics of a particular situation to determine their applicability to that situation (Sue, 2000).

enculturation: the acquisition of cultural knowledge that allows one to function as a member of a particular society.

ethnicity: a construct used to describe group identification with a particular country or heritage.

ethnographic approach: a strategy for data collection using observation, interview, and other qualitative methods.

ethnography: the study and detailed description of human groups using direct observation and interview.

explanatory models: the ways in which persons understand sickness or unwanted conditions.

fact-centered: an approach to teaching cultural competence focused on learning about the beliefs and behaviors of specific ethnic groups.

focus: the predetermined set of interests one brings to interactions.

foreign language translator: an individual who speaks two languages and can translate from one to the other and back.

gender identity: an individual's identification as either male or female, usually based on genetic and physical characteristics and reinforced by learned behavior.

genetic adaptation: changes in biological characteristics to facilitate survival in a particular location, thought to be an evolutionary response to environmental circumstances.

group spokesperson: a religious authority, tribal elder, or public figure associated with a recognized organization who represents a member of an ethnic or social group, usually by making pronouncements on the ethical dimensions of an issue.

harmony with nature: a value orientation found in some cultures that suggests that humans must live in harmony with natural phenomena.

health: absence of sickness or presence of desired abilities and quality of life.

hot-cold belief system: folk medical system in which certain substances in the environment and the individual are classified as hot or cold and have specific illness-causing or curative properties related to that classification.

individuality: social relationship structure defined by degree of autonomy of the individual.

innovation: culture change through development of new technologies or ideas.

inquiry-centered approach: an approach to learning about culture that emphasizes asking questions and gathering information about the specific situation (Johnson, Hardt, & Kleinman, 1995).

insiders: members of a cultural group.

interactional moment: a point in time in the interaction between two or more individuals.

intercultural: across or among multiple cultures.

intracultural variability: difference among individuals within a group identified as representing a specific culture.

life as narrative: a perspective that holds that life is experienced primarily as an unfolding, and then as a remembered, story.

lineality: social relationship structure defined by biological and cultural relationship over time.

localization: culture always situated in personally meaningful, interactive locations.

mastery over nature: a value orientation found in some cultures that suggests that humans can and should gain control of natural phenomena.

member checking: a form of triangulation in which the "other" data source is the client him- or herself.

moxabustion: therapeutic burning as a form of cure for such ailments as malaria, hepatitis, and abdominal problems used by an array of cultures.

multicultural: including or reflective of many cultures.

multiple subjectivities: a perspective on experience that holds that individuals may perceive a single event or experience in different ways (Rakos, 1999).

mutual cultural accommodation: the process by which individuals make modest adaptations in their behavior based on new knowledge from a previous contact with another culture.

normative behavior: behavior consistent with the beliefs, values, and expectations of a cultural group.

outsiders: those who are not members of a cultural group.

palliative care: care to promote comfort rather than to cure illness.

participant observation: a process by which an ethnographer or fieldworker lives in a community and participates as much as possible in its routines while constantly observing.

personality: "an individual's characteristic pattern of thought, emotion, and behavior, together with the psychological mechanisms—hidden or not—behind those patterns" (Funder, 1997, pp. 1-2).

placebo effect: improvement in a health condition as a result of provision of a substance or procedure believed to be inert (i.e., to have no observable chemical or physical effect).

qualitative interviewing: interviewing that makes use of ethnographic methods to obtain rich, detailed description of the subject.

qualitative methods: methods such as interviewing and observation used to gather detailed, extensive, and in-depth information about a situation.

quality of life: evaluative assessment of life in terms of the extent to which it is perceived as positive.

race: a construct typically used to describe apparent biological differences among groups.

regulation: a process of managing individual conduct by providing normative messages in communication.

rite of passage: ritual associated with the life cycle of a single individual.

rites of intensification: rituals resulting from or commemorating changes in the environment designed to confirm, strengthen, or display group membership or identity.

ritual: a patterned, repeated, formalized behavior engaged in by individuals but sanctioned by groups.

role conflict: the tension that arises from occupying several roles that carry incompatible expectations.

rules approach: a method for describing a culture through identification of the ways in which people view reality, make distinctions among categories of things, and make decisions about right courses of action.

scientific-mindedness: a mindset that emphasizes generating hypotheses about situations and gathering data to help confirm or refute the hypotheses (Sue, 2000).

shaman: a type of specialized healer commonly found in many traditional cultures in North and South America.

shamanic path: a way of seeing and knowing that which is hidden from ordinary members of a community but revealed to a shaman.

social constructivists: those who believe in a psychological relativism suggesting that perceptions of individuals and individuality are culturally defined rather than biologically dictated.

social role: the behavior expected as appropriate for a specific status position in a particular situation.

social structure: the relationship of various status positions in a society.

society: an organization of people.

status: a position in society with certain rights and obligations.

stereotype: a generalization or categorization about a particular group based on some common feature like gender or physical appearance.

stretching: a sense of being challenged to change some cultural assumptions and practices in response to encounters with individuals of differing identities (Kim, 1996).

subjective well-being: individual perceptions of positive events and level of happiness based on personal, internal experience.

subjugation to nature: a value orientation found in some cultures that suggests that humans are controlled by the natural world.

triangulation: a mechanism by which various information sources are checked against each other to confirm interpretations.

trustworthiness: when referring to qualitative data, the dependability, credibility, transferability, and applicability of the information gathered.

underground practice: a mechanism by which health care professionals adhere to organizational dicta while finding ways to meet client needs that do not conform to those dicta (Mattingly, 1998).

universal: cultural institution or belief shared by almost all groups.

value orientation: a predisposition toward a particular set or kind of values.

values: people's beliefs about the goals or way of life that is desirable for themselves and their society (Peoples & Bailey, 1997, p. 22).

vantage: any observing mind's specific point of view with physical, psychological, and cultural dimensions that restrict how much can be observed at any moment.

vantage effects: the ways in which vantage alters one's perception of reality.

world view: the way in which people "perceive and interpret reality and events, including their images of themselves and how they relate to the world around them" (Peoples & Bailey, 1997, p. 26).

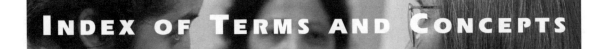

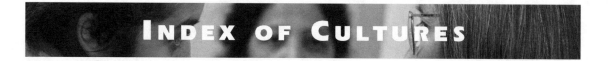

INDEX OF CULTURES

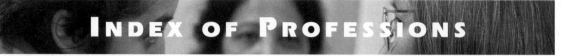

INDEX OF PROFESSIONS

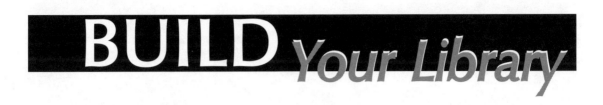

BUILD *Your Library*

This book and many others on numerous different topics are available from SLACK Incorporated. For further information or a copy of our latest catalog, contact us at:

Professional Book Division
SLACK Incorporated
6900 Grove Road
Thorofare, NJ 08086 USA
Telephone: 1-856-848-1000
1-800-257-8290
Fax: 1-856-853-5991
E-mail: orders@slackinc.com
www.slackbooks.com

We accept most major credit cards and checks or money orders in US dollars drawn on a US bank. Most orders are shipped within 72 hours.

Contact us for information on recent releases, forthcoming titles, and bestsellers. If you have a comment about this title or see a need for a new book, direct your correspondence to the Editorial Director at the above address.

Thank you for your interest and we hope you found this work beneficial.